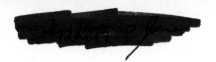

D1411698

THE BASIC NEUROLOGY
OF SPEECH AND
LANGUAGE

MICHAEL L. E. ESPIR

FRCP

Honorary Consultant Neurologist, Charing Cross
and Northwick Park Hospitals
Honorary Lecturer, Institute of Neurology,
National Hospital, Queen Square, London
Lecturer in Neurology, National Hospital's
College of Speech Sciences
Principal Medical Officer, Civil Service
Medical Advisory Service

AND

F. CLIFFORD ROSE

FRCP

Physician in Charge, Department of Neurology,
Charing Cross Hospital
Consultant Neurologist, Medical Ophthalmology Unit,
St Thomas' Hospital
Member of the Academy of Aphasia

THIRD EDITION

BLACKWELL SCIENTIFIC PUBLICATIONS
OXFORD LONDON EDINBURGH
MELBOURNE BOSTON

© 1970, 1976, 1983 by
Blackwell Scientific Publications
Editorial offices:
Osney Mead, Oxford OX2 0EL
8 John Street, London WC1N 2ES
9 Forrest Road, Edinburgh EH1 2QH
52 Beacon Street, Boston,
    Massachusetts 02108, USA
99 Barry Street, Carlton
    Victoria 3053, Australia

First published 1970
Second edition 1976
Third edition 1983

Set by Charlton Graphics, Croydon
Printed and bound in Great Britain by
Billing & Sons Limited, Worcester

DISTRIBUTORS

USA
  Blackwell Mosby Book Distributors
  11830 Westline Industrial Drive
  St Louis, Missouri 63141

Canada
  Blackwell Mosby Book Distributors
  120 Melford Drive, Scarborough
  Ontario M1B 2X4

Australia
  Blackwell Scientific Book Distributors
  31 Advantage Road, Highett
  Victoria 3190

British Library
Cataloguing in Publication Data

Espir, M. L. E.
  The basic neurology of speech and
  language
  1. Speech, Disorders of
  I. Rose, F. C.
  616.85′5   RC423

ISBN 0–632–01068–1

CONTENTS

PART 2

PREFACE TO THE THIRD EDITION

During the last decade there have been important and exciting advances in neurology, not only in methods of investigation and treatment, but also in our knowledge of the mechanism of production of certain diseases. Nevertheless the fundamentals of the subject have changed little since the previous edition of *The Basic Neurology of Speech*. Although many contributions in the linguistic and psychological fields have been made, the purpose of this book remains as before to provide a basic text of the neurology of speech and language disorders. Detailed descriptions of the relevant aspects are given for those whose main interest is in the speech disorders and who require a working knowledge of the neurological diseases which affect speech and language.

This third edition contains additional chapters and expanded sections about conditions which were neglected or dealt with only briefly in our previous editions, and also include updated accounts where advances have occurred.

This book is not meant to replace textbooks on neurology and aphasia but rather to be complementary, for those who require basic knowledge about the causes and pathological backgrounds of the clinical conditions likely to be encountered in practice. This explains the uneven coverage of various topics and why we do not attempt to give a comprehensive account of conditions that do not affect speech.

The same format as in the second edition has been maintained. Part 1 includes descriptions of the brain and its functions with details of the disturbances of speech and language and the other main manifestations of brain disorders. The chapters on dementia and epilepsy are particularly relevant, the latter having been revised and enlarged in the hope of overcoming the many misconceptions and difficulties in understanding this subject. Part 2 outlines the pathological conditions of special relevance in the production of speech and language disorders. The need and demand for more detailed clinical accounts of the neurological diseases with the highest prevalence has led to the addition of chapters on Parkinson's disease and multiple sclerosis, strokes being dealt with under the heading of vascular disorders. We considered it necessary also to add a separate chapter on motor neurone disease to try and clarify the clinical types resulting from involvement of upper and lower motor neurones either separately or in combination.

Considerable interest and research continues to be focussed on unravelling the causes and cure of these diseases, but in the meantime the technological advances in electronics is leading to the increasing development of communication aids and devices which will help the speech-impaired. As more sophisticated microprocessor based aids become available, there is an urgent need for information regarding the prevalence of severe speech disorders which are most likely to benefit. It is hoped that this book will also help those in the microprocessor field who wish to have a concise and clear account of the neurology of speech and language.

Our aim has been to make the relevant aspects of neurology easier to understand for those who need an introduction and working knowledge of the subject. Although intended primarily for speech therapists, this description of the neurological disorders affecting speech and language should also be helpful for medical students, nurses and other paramedical groups (e.g. psychologists, physiotherapists and occupational therapists).

We are very pleased to acknowledge our debt to colleagues for helpful discussions, particularly to Alison Perry, chief speech therapist at the Charing Cross Hospital, for her comments and suggestions. Special thanks are again due to Mrs Patricia Espir for typing the manuscript, Mr Brian Armitage for the index, and the publishers for the production of this book.

PREFACE TO SECOND EDITION

During the 6 years since the publication of the first edition, there has been a considerable increase in the world literature on speech and language disorders, and also a growing interest in the field of neurolinguistics. It is not the authors' aim with this book to provide a comprehensive review but rather to present in simplified form the neurological aspects of speech. In this edition there is a rearrangement of chapters and the book is now divided into two parts.

In Part 1, the brain, its functions and their derangements, and the various types of speech and language disorders are described.

Part 2 gives a concise account of brain disorders which can influence speech and language. Only those anatomical, physiological and pathological details required for the understanding of basic neurology have been included, and reference to larger text books will be needed for more comprehensive accounts of neurological disorders. However, we hope that this small volume will make this difficult subject more readily understandable for those concerned with the neurological aspects of communication.

Few books satisfy both students and specialist. The first edition, being based on our lectures to schools of speech therapy and on subsequent experience as examiners in neurology for the College of Speech Therapists and University of Newcastle upon Tyne, seemed to have filled a gap for student and practising speech therapists. As a basic text, the book has to be reasonably inexpensive and act as a guide to the more specialised works referred to in the bibliography.

We are grateful for the constructive criticism of the reviewers of the previous edition, and for helpful discussions with our neurologist and speech therapist colleagues. Many suggestions have been incorporated into this edition and chapters have been enlarged, e.g. memory and amnesia (Chapter 3), the part of laryngeal reflexes in the mechanism of stammering (Chapter 8) and dysphonia (Chapter 12). A chapter has been added on trauma in view of its importance as a cause of speech disorders.

We are grateful to the Librarian at the Nottingham General

Hospital for checking the bibliography and also to the Departments of Medical Illustration at the Nottingham General and Charing Cross Hospitals for help with the diagrams.

We are also indebted once again to our secretaries for their help with the manuscript, to Mr Brian Armitage for preparing the index and to the publishers for the production of this book.

PREFACE TO FIRST EDITION

There is a vast literature on the many disciplines with which speech is concerned, but this book is intended as a simple presentation of the neurological approach to its anatomy, physiology and pathology. Although based on courses of lectures given by the authors in three of the schools of speech therapy in Great Britain, it should prove helpful not only to speech therapists, both for their final examinations and for practice afterwards, but also to medical students and others in disciplines concerned with communication (e.g. paediatrics, psychiatry, psychology, phonetics and linguistics).

The neurological mechanisms of speech and its disorders are complex and because of our pragmatic simplification a selected bibliography is given.

It is a pleasure to acknowledge our indebtedness to our teachers and colleagues who are too numerous to mention individually. We are particularly grateful to Professor W. Ritchie Russell and the Clarendon Press for permission to quote from the book *Traumatic Aphasia*, and also to Dr Macdonald Critchley and the late Lord Brain for their teaching and literature.

We also thank the authors and publishers who have given permission for the reproduction of the illustrations acknowledged in the text. We are grateful to Dr Paul Millac for reading the proofs and making helpful suggestions, and to Mr B. Armitage, Librarian at the Charing Cross Hospital Medical School for preparing the index.

Our thanks are due to Mrs Vanessa Dussek and Mrs Patricia Espir for their patience in typing and retyping the chapters, and to the Department of Medical Illustration of Charing Cross Hospital for help with diagrams.

PART 1

CHAPTER 1

INTRODUCTION

Speech is unique to man. It can be defined as a system of communication in which thoughts are expressed and understood by using acoustic symbols. They are produced by the vibration of the vocal cords in the larynx (phonation), caused by the flow of air (respiration) and given final form by movements of the lips, tongue and palate (articulation).

Speech refers to verbal symbols, but language includes the non-verbal aspects of communication, for example—gesticulation, gesture and pantomime, each of which is different. Gesticulation is the associated muscular movement which emphasises speech. Pantomime is a method of communication in which spoken language is replaced by acting, and may include a series of gestures, each of which conveys a single meaning. Language includes all systems of communication, not only speech but the expression and understanding of written words, signs, gestures and music.

THE DEVELOPMENT OF SPEECH

It is important to realise firstly the comparatively late acquirement of speech in biological history (phylogenetic development), and secondly to understand how an individual person learns to speak (ontogenetic development).

Phylogenetic development

The age of the planet on which we live has been estimated as 4000 million years. Life in its earliest form started about 1000 million years ago. An animal capable of making a noise (i.e. possessing a jointed larynx) came into existence 200 million years ago, but true and false vocal cords with the formation of a cochlea did not take place until perhaps 50 million years ago.

Although some animals, for example, the cock, hawk and rat

3

make signals, and apes chatter and lions roar, these sounds are inborn, species-characteristic and limited to a specific reaction. The talking of parrots is mimicry and not speech in the scientific sense since there is no question of the bird formulating thoughts into words or understanding the sounds it utters. The 'language' of birds is in fact limited to communicating their desire for food, sexual needs, warnings of danger or mimicry, whereas human language covers an infinite number of thoughts, abstract as well as concrete. Questions can be asked and answered allowing an exchange of ideas and arguments, and humans also have the unique privilege of telling lies, believing or disbelieving. Although the faculty of speech is inborn, individual language has to be learnt.

There are several hypotheses as to how man acquired speech. Max Müller described the following:
1   The 'Ding-dong' theory—suggesting that there is an inherent connection between words and the things they stand for.
2   The 'Bow-wow' theory—suggesting that speech arose out of onomatopoeic sounds.
3   The 'Pooh-pooh' theory— indicating that by involuntary sounds and interjection, speech was acquired like the 'speech' of lower animals and birds.
4   The 'Yo-heave-ho' theory—suggesting that man began to learn to speak from the sounds associated with communal physical effort.
Early speech consisted of cries of emotion (e.g. fear, joy, anger) and these corresponded to animal sound signals. Curses and exclamations lack the distinctive features of human speech since they may be uttered involuntarily and are automatic expressions of the emotions. Some of these interjections are conventionally described as 'whew', 'ah', 'urgh', 'humph'.

The earliest man of which we have evidence (Java man) lived about one million years ago. A more developed creature (Heidelberg man) appeared half a million years ago, Neanderthal man about 150 000 years ago, and Cromagnon man about 50 000 years ago. Man began to speak as soon as he used tools (i.e. during the first Pleistocene period): the cooperation of individuals is needed both for speech and the use of tools and probably the first role of speech was to control behaviour.

Man did not give up his nomadic life and develop agriculture until 7000 BC, whereas the first writing of which we have evidence is approximately 4000 BC: the Samarians of Mesopotamia were writing 3500 years before the birth of Christ. Speech, then, is a recent development in the history of the world and its life.

Ontogenetic development of speech

Speech is acquired by the process of learning, which may be defined as the change in behaviour and perception of an organism as a consequence of its experience. A baby produces sound by crying as soon as it is born and, after a month, the cry becomes differentiated so that a mother appreciates its particular significance. As early as 2 months, an infant recognises the human voice, and soon after begins babbling: this is an essential part in the development of speech since it is a means of autostimulation (auditory feedback): the baby will stop babbling with any auditory stimulus—particularly if spoken to. At 6 months, the infant will distinguish between affectionate and scolding terms, and about this time the babbling becomes rhythmic (lalling). At about 9 months of age the child recognises familiar words and says 'Mama' and 'Dada'. It repeats words it hears—echolalia or psittacism, ('psittakos'—a parrot). The child loses nearly all the babbling sounds when it begins to articulate, and some children pass through a mute period between the babbling and language learning periods. In all languages, vowels are learned before consonants, the first vowel learned is an 'a', and the first consonant is an 'm'.

At 12 months of age, there will be a response to simple commands, and by 18 months the infant will acquire several words, many of which are peculiar to the child (idioglossia) but about 10–20 of these are meaningful. Although the learning of speech is relatively slow in the first 18 months, it is rapid for the next year, so that by the age of 2½ years the child can say two-word phrases. The rate of learning slows off at the age of 2½ years, the child acquiring about 500 new words each year and fully acquired speech—involving the use of sentences—comes gradually during the next few years.

The rapidity of learning depends not only on intelligence, but on the stimulation to speak (e.g. the home atmosphere and the social class of the parents). An only child is more likely to develop speech earlier than twins; the child of bilingual parents and a child in an orphanage are often slower than average.

The laborious learning of words, movements and reactions during early childhood depends on a system of repetitions and copying, trial and error. When the infant learns his first word, he has been listening to sounds of both himself and his mother; both use their personal pleasure as a facilitating mechanism, so that the sound is repeated in order to experience the pleasure again. When a child says 'Dada' he is repeating what he hears and then he correlates this with the seeing of a man; this necessitates remembering what the man looks like, and experiencing a feeling of familiarity and pleasure at the sight. The first process of repeating sounds soon becomes associated with the receptive systems, especially vision. The various sensations, including those from the muscles of the mouth and larynx, are essential for the registration of the neuronal patterns required to make the various noises that result in speech. The subsequent development of vocabulary and grammar is an elaboration of the more fundamental mechanism of registration. Learning to read and write, and correct spelling, involves many complex processes as does the capacity to name an object. Writing and reading are then learnt according to a programme and this capacity for learning is developed so that further knowledge can be superimposed. The neurological mechanisms depend partly on the repetition of previous responses; this is closely concerned with memory, which in its simplest form is the ability to repeat or recall a previous stimulus.

Animals learn to respond to sights, sounds and other sensations with motor reactions which may include making a noise; man has learned to produce a great variety of noises in relation to different objects, activities and feelings; in doing this, he uses highly specialised parts of his brain. Language and speech, as well as the related faculties of memory, learning and calculation are dependent on brain mechanisms which are integrated in, and controlled by, the cerebral hemispheres.

Further Reading

BRAIN W.R. (1965) *Speech Disorders*, 2e. Butterworths, London.

CRITCHLEY M. (1975) *Silent Language*. Butterworths, London.

DE CECCO J.P. (1964) *The Psychology of Language, Thought and Instruction*. Holt, Rinehart and Winston, London.

LOCK S., CAPLAN D. & KELLAR L. (1973) *A Study in Neurolinguistics*. C.C. Thomas, Springfield, Illinois.

MASON S.E. (ed.) (1963) *Signs, Signals and Symbols*. Methuen, London.

CHAPTER 2
THE BRAIN AND ITS FUNCTIONS

The brain is the most complicated organ of the body. It is composed of a complex network of nerve cells and fibres, requiring a rich blood supply (see Chapter 17) so that adequate oxygen, glucose, vitamins etc, are made available for metabolism. Restriction of these requirements will impair brain function and destruction of the nerve cells will lead to irreversible disorders.

Embryologically the anterior end of the central nervous system is modified into three parts, viz. the fore-brain, mid-brain and hind-brain. With development these parts increase in size and complexity, so that an adult human brain consists of many folded areas (gyri) with fissures in between (sulci). This convolutional pattern enables man to have the maximum amount of cerebral cortex in the smallest possible volume.

The surface of the brain (cortex) comprises the grey matter, which contains the nerve *cells* (neurones). This covers the underlying white matter which consists mainly of nerve *fibres.* In addition to the nerve cells and their fibres, the brain substance also contains connective tissue cells. These are of three types: astrocytes, oligodendrocytes and microglia. There are also aggregations of neurones (nuclei) forming the basal ganglia which lie in the depths of each cerebral hemisphere. The cerebral hemispheres are joined together by the corpus callosum and each is connected with the brain stem by the cerebral peduncles. The brain stem has three parts: mid-brain, pons and medulla (or bulb).

The cerebellum consists of right and left cerebellar hemispheres, joined in the mid line by the vermis. Each cerebellar hemisphere is connected to the corresponding side of the brain stem by three cerebellar peduncles: superior (brachium conjunctivum), middle (brachium pontis) and inferior (restiform body).

Each cerebral hemisphere consists of frontal, parietal, temporal and occipital lobes (see Fig. 1). The central (Rolandic) fissure separates the frontal from the parietal lobe. The lateral (Sylvian) fissure demarcates the upper part of the temporal lobe. The occipital lobe

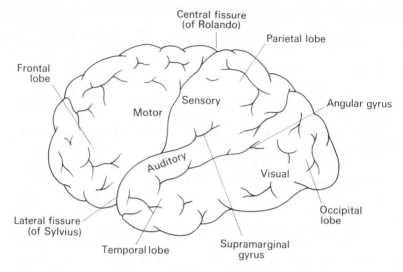

Fig. 1 Diagram of the lateral surface of the left cerebral hemisphere.

is the posterior part of the hemisphere, containing the calcarine (visual) cortex. Many of the main gyri are named and the whole cortex has been divided into anatomical regions, numbered as Brodmann's areas.

The phrenologists considered that the fissures divided the brain into regions which were concerned with personality characteristics, for example, intelligence, memory and piety. These attempts to localise specific function to certain anatomical areas conflicted with the view that the brain was an amorphous organ whose cells, like the cells of the liver, could function in many capacities. Localisation of speech function within the brain was suggested by Broca in 1861, and subsequent observations including experiments using electrical stimulation have shown that other important functions are controlled by specific parts of the brain. Thus the cerebral control of movements is located in the precentral gyrus which is the main motor area. The postcentral gyrus represents sensory functions; the visual cortex is in the occipital lobe. There are also so-called non-committed areas of the brain, for example in the frontal lobes, containing association fibres so that the brain can function as a whole.

THE SPEECH AREA

The surface markings of the area of the dominant cerebral hemi-sphere controlling speech and language functions are shown in Fig. 2. This includes the lowermost part of the precentral gyrus (Broca's area) and postcentral gyrus, the supramarginal and angular gyri, the inferior parietal gyri and upper part of the temporal lobe (Wernicke's area). The disorders of speech due to lesions in this area are described in Chapter 5. The concept of *cerebral dominance* is discussed in Chapter 4.

THE FRONTAL LOBES

The precentral gyrus in each cerebral hemisphere contains the motor cortex, in which the large motor nerve cells (Betz cells) are situated. The face is represented by the lowermost part in the inferior frontal region, there is a large area for the hand and upper limb in the middle, and the leg area is uppermost (viz. in the para-sagittal region) and extends over the medial surface of the hemi-sphere. The area anterior to the precentral gyrus is called the pre-motor cortex, which covers a large association area for the control of motor function.

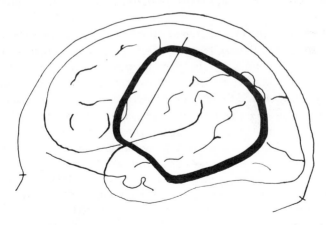

Fig. 2 The thick line indicates the limits of the area of the brain within which a small wound will cause aphasia (W.R. Russell 1963). The speech area thus lies within this and includes Broca's and Wernicke's areas. (Reproduced by permission of the author and the *Lancet*.)

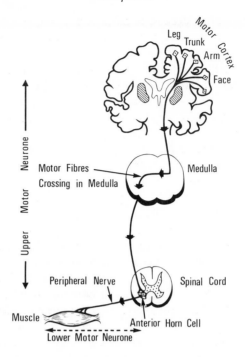

Fig. 3 Diagram of upper and lower neurones. (Redrawn from *Neurology* 3e, by E.R. Bickerstaff (1978). Hodder and Stoughton, London.)

Fibres from the motor cells of all parts of the motor cortex (see Fig. 3) penetrate the depths of the cerebral hemisphere in the corona radiata, coming closer together to pass through the internal capsule; this lies between the lenticular nucleus laterally and the caudate nucleus and thalamus medially. In the internal capsule, the fibres subserving the face area are in the front, the leg area posteriorly and the arm and trunk fibres in between. The fibres then descend through the cerebral peduncles, mid-brain and pons. In the brain stem most of the cortico*bulbar* fibres cross to the opposite side and terminate in synapses (see page 53) with the *motor nuclei of the cranial nerves*. Likewise the majority of cortico*spinal* fibres cross (decussate) to form the pyramids, and then descend in the lateral columns of the spinal cord as the pyramidal (corticospinal) tracts, terminating in synapses with the *anterior horn cells of the spinal cord*. This is the first part of the motor pathway, the upper motor neurone (UMN). It thus extends from the motor cells of the frontal cortex, either via the corticobulbar fibres to the synapses with the cells of the motor nuclei of the cranial nerves in the medulla, or via the corticospinal fibres to the synapses with the anterior horn cells of the spinal cord. The upper motor neurones transmit the impulses from the cerebral hemispheres which initiate, associate and control voluntary and automatic muscular action and reaction. They are linked in the cerebral hemispheres by the association areas with the other parts of the brain which receive the sensory, visual and auditory stimuli. Integration of stimuli received by, and emanating from, all parts of the brain allows co-ordinated physical and mental reactions, and the separation of functions for the purpose of description is artificial. It may also be fallacious to draw conclusions about the normal functioning of the brain from a study of the effects of damage to localised areas. (Comparison can be made with an electrical circuit where damage to the battery or generating system will have an effect on all points and connections, whereas damage to a single wire will have very different effects depending upon its situation in the circuit and its relation to other points, for example, whether connected in series or parallel.)

Bilateral representation

The majority of the corticobulbar fibres from each cerebral hemisphere cross over to the opposite side in the brain stem, but not all do, a small proportion remaining uncrossed. As a result of this arrangement, the motor nuclei of the cranial nerves in the brain stem—with the exception of the lower part of the facial nucleus—receive impulses from both crossed and uncrossed corticobulbar fibres which gives them bilateral cerebral representation. So when the corticobulbar fibres from one cerebral hemisphere are damaged, function of the cranial nerves may be maintained by the uncrossed fibres from the unaffected hemisphere. This explains why hemiplegic patients usually have no paralysis of the upper part of the face, nor of the palate or tongue. Movements such as frowning, wrinkling the forehead and breathing are normally done by simultaneous symmetrical contractions of the muscles on both sides, each side being controlled by both cerebral hemispheres, so that paralysis of these functions does not result from a unilateral cerebral lesion involving the corticobulbar fibres from that hemisphere (for further details about this, see Chapter 7, pages 61).

Other frontal lobe functions

Personality, temperament, emotional control and behaviour are dependent upon mechanisms in the frontal lobes, and these may become disturbed if either or both of the frontal lobes become damaged or diseased. The frontal lobes are often considered to be the seat of the mind and intelligence, but intellectual function is dependent upon integration of the whole cerebral cortex. Normal behaviour depends largely on a balance between initiative and self control, and the ability to act appropriately has come to be part of everyday life and social necessity. The primitive instincts of a child normally become inhibited by conditioning and, with maturity, customs and etiquette are learnt so that impulses, emotions and actions are suppressed to conform with the requirements of the environment.

Voluntary control of movements of the head and neck and eye are also associated with frontal lobe function, as is control of the bladder and sexual functions.

Frontal lobe syndromes

Patients with frontal lobe disorders manifest disinhibition, with inadequately controlled, aggressive or antisocial behaviour, as well as dementia (see Chapter 13), deterioration of personality and intellect, slowness of thought and loss of initiative. The mental changes resulting from frontal lobe lesions include defects of emotional control; there is a tendency to laugh childishly or inappropriately, with inability to realise the true seriousness of situations, for example, lack of insight into the gravity of medical disability. Changes in mood range from the feeling of well-being or excessive cheerfulness (euphoria) which is inappropriate and pathological, to mania; alternatively the patient becomes depressed, miserable and melancholic without adequate reason.

Lesions in the motor area will cause weakness of the opposite side of the body, i.e. the face, arm or leg, according to the situation and extent of the lesion. The terms *hemiparesis* or *hemiplegia* are used to describe respectively weakness or paralysis of one half of the body (i.e. face, arm and leg); *monoplegia* means paralysis of one limb, either arm or leg (see Chapter 7).

THE PARIETAL LOBES

The parietal lobes are the main receiving areas for sensory impulses and stimuli. Parts of the body are represented in the contralateral sensory cortex of the postcentral gyrus in the same way as on the motor side. The sensory impulses travel from the end organs in the skin, muscles, joints and other tissues of the body and are conveyed proximally in centripetal fashion via the sensory (spinal and cranial) nerves. From the dorsal root ganglia, the fibres of the posterior nerve roots enter the spinal cord and form the main sensory tracts, which pass up via the brain stem to the first receiving station in the thalamus. The impulses are then relayed from the thalamus through the posterior part of the internal capsule and radiate out to the appropriate parts of the sensory cortex.

Basic sensations such as touch pass to the postcentral gyrus, whereas impulses for finer discrimination and interpretation pass to the large area of the parietal lobe posterior to the postcentral gyrus. These finer discriminative functions are concerned with size, shape and consistency of substances which are felt and allow differentiation of complicated sensations, appreciation of the sense of position of the opposite side of the body, and the location of particular parts of the body in space. This is a highly developed function which becomes automatic, so that the position and movement of a hand is known both in relation to a given object and also in relation to other parts of the body. Orientation in space and appreciation of the body-image (see page 21) are dependent upon the function of the association areas of the parietal region. These are linked with the visual cortex in the occipital region and performance of many manoeuvres is improved by seeing.

Parietal lobe syndromes

Damage to the sensory pathways or receiving areas in one parietal lobe will cause a contralateral hemianaesthesia, i.e. impairment of sensation on the opposite side of the body. If the lesion is localised, the sensory loss may be limited—e.g. to the hand or leg. Parietal lobe lesions may also cause various types of apraxia and agnosia, disorientation and disturbances of the body image (see Chapter 3) and a homonymous hemianopia if the optic radiation is involved (see page 15).

THE TEMPORAL LOBES

A large part of the temporal lobe of the dominant cerebral hemi-sphere is concerned with speech, particularly the middle zone of the upper temporal convolution (Wernicke's area). This forms part of the main auditory-receptive centre for the assimilation and inter-pretation of sounds required for the understanding of speech. The medial part of each temporal lobe includes the uncus, hippocampus and amygdaloid body which are concerned with the senses of *smell and taste* and with *memory* (see Chapter 12). The hippocampus is linked with the mamillary bodies (*corpora mamillaria*) via the fornix of the corpus callosum, which also forms a connection with the hippocampus of the opposite temporal lobe.

Lesions confined to the temporal lobe cause no motor or sensory changes on the opposite side of the body but may involve the optic radiation and produce contralateral homonymous visual field defects (see Fig. 4). The anterior 5–6 cm of one temporal lobe can be removed surgically (temporal lobectomy) without any obvious clinical sequelae.

THE OCCIPITAL LOBES

These contain the calcarine (visual) cortex. A complete lesion on one side will give a homonymous hemianopia on the opposite side (see Fig. 4c). Partial lesions of one occipital lobe will cause congruous defects or scotomata in the homonymous visual fields of various shapes, according to the exact extent of the lesion.

THE OPTIC RADIATION

The fibres forming this part of the visual pathway lie deep in the temporal and parietal lobes and convey impulses from the lateral geniculate body on each side to the visual cortex in the occipital lobe. A lesion of the temporal lobe may initially involve the lower part of the optic radiation as it passes round the temporal horn of the lateral ventricle and so cause contralateral homonymous *upper* quadrantic visual field defects (see Fig. 4a). A lesion of the parietal lobe may involve the upper part of the optic radiation and so cause contralateral homonymous *lower* quadrantic visual field defects (see Fig. 4b). If either temporal or parietal lobe lesions extend to involve the whole of the optic radiation, then a complete contralateral homonymous hemianopia will result (see Fig. 4c).

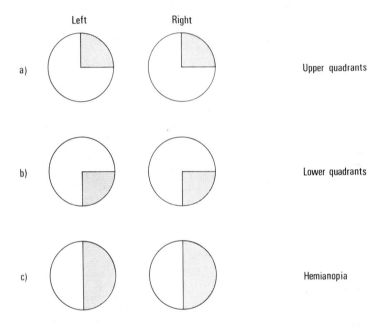

Fig. 4 Visual field defects (represented by shaded areas): (a) right homonymous upper quadrantic; (b) right homonymous lower quadrantic; (c) right homonymous hemianopia.

Further Reading

BOWSHER D. (1979) *Introduction to the Anatomy and Physiology of the Nervous System*, 4e. Blackwell Scientific Publications, Oxford.

BREWER C.V. (1961) *The Organisation of the Central Nervous System*. Heinemann, London.

CARTERETTE E.C. (ed.) (1966) Speech, Language and Communication; *Proceedings of the third conference on brain function*, November 1963. University of California Press, Berkeley.

CHERRY C. (1957) *On Human Communication*. Chapman and Hall, London.

LURIA A.R. (1973) *The Working Brain: An Introduction to Neuropsychology*. Penguin Books, Harmondsworth.

MATTHEWS B. (1968) *Introduction to Clinical Neurology*, 3e. E & S Livingstone, Edinburgh.

MILLIKAN C.H. & DARLEY F.I. (eds.) (1967) Conference on Brain Mechanisms underlying Speech and Language: *Proceedings of a Conference held at Princetown, NJ, 1965*. Grune and Stratton, New York.

NATHAN P. (1982) *The Nervous System*. Penguin Books 2e, Harmondsworth.

RUSSELL W.R. (1959) *Brain, Memory, Learning*. Clarendon Press, Oxford.

RUSSELL W.R. (1963) Some Anatomical Aspects of Aphasia. *Lancet* i, 1173–7.

CHAPTER 3
APRAXIA AND AGNOSIA

APRAXIA

The ability to perform purposeful movements and complicated skills is gradually learned by practice and experience; these motor activities are organised and stored by the association areas of the frontal and parietal lobes. Apraxia is the loss of skill or ability to perform specific actions at will or command, yet the same movements can be performed spontaneously. There is no paralysis and the individual muscles can participate in other actions. The causative lesion involves the relevant association areas controlling the pattern or plan of manoeuvres, and interferes with the performance of movements initiated by the corresponding part of the motor cortex, although the fibres forming the main motor pathway remain intact.

In general, the more recently acquired actions are lost first, so that in mild cases the less complicated and primitive skills are preserved. In severe forms the patient regresses to a state comparable to infancy with incoordinate movements affecting actions such as walking or standing. These movements, performed automatically in adult life, are based on the concept of 'kinetic engrams' and the disturbances of these have been called limb-kinetic, innervatory or cortical apraxia.

Ideomotor apraxia. This is the term suggested when the kinetic engrams are present. The patient has no difficulty in formulating the idea of the act which he wishes to carry out but finds himself unable to execute it. For example, a patient with a left cerebral lesion but no hemiplegia, may be able to hold objects and write with the right hand, yet be unable to perform certain actions such as saluting or polishing. If he is able to do so with the left hand, this clearly demonstrates that he understands the request, he knows what has to be done but cannot convert the idea into the required action with the right hand.

17

Ideational apraxia. This occurs when the conception of the movement is faulty and affects both sides of the body. It is most obvious with complex manoeuvres such as putting on a jacket, but may also interfere with even simpler movements to order—for example if the patient is asked to brush his hair. In severe forms, ideational apraxia is combined with ideomotor apraxia.

Loss of the ability to put on or take off clothes in an orderly fashion or without becoming muddled (*dressing apraxia*) may occur as an isolated disability but is often associated with failure to construct models from blocks or letters with matches (*constructional apraxia*).

Apraxia may be restricted to the face, lips or tongue, described as oral-facial apraxia, the patient being unable to make a frown or grimace when told to or even imitate one when shown. Protrusion of the tongue when requested may be impossible yet the movement may be done automatically when licking the lips. Facial apraxia (apraxia of facial movements) may occur either with or without disturbance of speech, and in some cases dysarthria is due to facial apraxia. If there is apraxia for the movements required for articulation, this is articulatory apraxia or apraxic dysarthria, which may or not be accompanied by bilateral apraxia of the face. Facial apraxia and dysarthria are also common accompaniments of Broca's motor aphasia (see Chapter 5). It has also been suggested that Brocas's aphasia may be an apraxia of speech, but this has caused confusion amongst aphasiologists, and until the physiological and neuropsychological aspects of this complicated problem have been resolved, we restrict the use of the terms apraxia and dysarthria to non-linguistic disorders of movement and articulation, even though in severe cases they may accompany and be part of the problem of motor aphasia.

Constructional apraxia may interfere with drawing or writing, and may be distinguished from other types of dysgraphia resulting from a specific defect of language.

Apraxia is thus a motor disability, without paralysis and without failure to understand what is requested. If there is also an element of agnosia (see below) there is then a failure to recognise the nature or purpose of the object for which the movements are required; in dressing apraxia, the patient may be unable to relate the spatial forms of his garments to that of his body, and in constructional apraxia the patient may be unaware of the inadequacy of his achievement, indicating defective recognition both of the model and the copy.

The site of the lesion causing apraxia is usually the postcentral area of the parietal lobe and its connections with the motor cortex in the frontal lobe, either on the same side or with both sides through the corpus callosum. Constructional apraxia may be caused by a lesion in either hemisphere, but dressing apraxia usually results from a lesion of the non-dominant parietal lobe.

AGNOSIA

The ability to interpret sensory stimuli which are conveyed to the brain from the special senses (e.g. visual and auditory) and from other parts of the body (e.g. touch) is a function of the cerebral hemispheres. The cortex of the temporal, parietal and occipital lobes are mainly concerned with the processes of recognition or perception of sensory stimuli (gnosis). This implies that the crude sensory stimuli acquire significance by collation with previous experiences stored as memories in the appropriate association areas.

Agnosia, a term first introduced by Freud in 1891, means a loss of this ability to recognise these sensory experiences; it is a defect of perception due to a disorder of cerebral mechanisms. The lesions causing the defects involve localised areas of the cerebral cortex and their association areas, the primary sensory pathways being intact. The various types of agnosia depend on the sensory modality involved.

Visual agnosia

Visual agnosia was called 'imperception' by Hughlings Jackson and various types are now described.

Visual object agnosia is the inability to recognise objects seen, this failure not being attributable to defects of vision or to general intellectual impairment. Not only is there failure to recognise an object but also what the object is used for (cf: nominal aphasia, in which the object cannot be named but its nature or use can often be described). A patient with visual agnosia is usually able to name the object if allowed to feel it. The lesion responsible for visual object agnosia is thought to be in the cortex of the 2nd and 3rd occipital convolutions or possibly in the splenium of the corpus callosum, through which pass fibres linking the visual cortex of the two hemispheres.

Visual object agnosia is sometimes associated with tactile agnosia, alexia, constructional apraxia and Gerstmann's syndrome (see page 22).

Dyslexia (see Chapters 6 and 9) may also be a type of visual agnosia, when the patterns produced by letters, words, numbers or music fail to be recognised or understood. The meaning must be stored in order to obtain the sequence of what follows. A homonymous hemianopia due to lesions of the optic radiation may also cause difficulty with reading; but the difficulties due to defects of the visual fields and of visual acuity differ from dyslexia which concerns the problems of using and understanding visual symbol patterns. The visual pathways of the brain play a large part in language, learning, memory and thought; congenitally blind patients develop speech mechanisms differently (Critchley 1953).

Spelling difficulties may also be due to disturbances of visual imagery due to lesions in the posterior parietal region.

Many other types of visual agnosia have been described. *Prosopagnosia* is a name given to the failure to recognise faces, normally well-known. *Simultanagnosia* is the failure to appreciate the meaning of a complex picture or recognise a combination of details although the individual elements are correctly recognised. This is also called visual extinction and indicates a lesion of the posterior temporal or parietal lobe. Visual inattention is the failure to see an object on one side when shown objects on both sides of the visual field simultaneously, there being no defect when each object is shown separately. *Agnosia for colours* has to be distinguished from nominal aphasia in which the colours are recognised but cannot be named. *Visual disorientation* may include defective visual localisation, loss of visual imagery, loss of stereoscopic vision and spatial agnosia. *Loss of topographical memory* may also occur independently of other forms of visual disorientation and of loss of memory for objects.

Auditory agnosia

In auditory agnosia, hearing is not impaired but there is an inability to recognise or distinguish the sounds which are heard due to a lesion of the left superior temporal convolution. With the eyes closed or covered, the patient cannot recognise familiar noises, such as the jingling of keys or coins. The loss of recognition of musical sounds is called *sensory amusia*. Failure to understand spoken speech (word deafness or receptive aphasia) may also be a form of auditory agnosia.

Tactile agnosia

Tactile agnosia, the failure to recognise objects by touch, is also called *astereognosis*. Sensation in the hands is otherwise normal, but the patient fails to recognise the shape, size or consistency of the object, which is placed in his hand without his being allowed to see it. Tactile agnosia may occur without visual agnosia, so that patients can then recognise by sight what they cannot recognise by feel. The lesion responsible is thought to be in the supramarginal gyrus of the parietal lobe, and there is evidence that in right handed persons bilateral tactile agnosia may be produced by a lesion in this area of the left cerebral hemisphere, suggesting that there may be dominance for tactile recognition.

The body image

The perception and recognition of movements of all parts of our body both in relation to each other and to the external environment are integrated so that we develop a body schema or awareness of our body image. Learning and memory mechanisms allow the use of previous experiences so that mental and physical performances become automatic or can be geared to changes in oneself or in the environment. This concept of the body image implies that storage, collating and selecting systems exist in the association areas, particularly of the parietal lobes.

Somatagnosia is the name given to disorders of the body schema; these include imperception or neglect of parts of the body (*autotopagnosia*) right-left disorientation (i.e. the inability to distinguish right from left) and denial of disability, e.g. unawareness of a hemiplegic limb (*anosognosia*). Another example is seen in some patients with complete cortical blindness who deny that they are blind but confabulate that they can see (*Anton's syndrome*).

The variety of possible defects, single and combined, is considerable. One such combination is *Gerstmann's syndrome*, viz: finger agnosia (an inability of the patient to recognise or identify his own fingers or those of the observer) right-left disorientation, agraphia and acaculia.

Site of lesions causing agnosia

Gerstmann's syndrome results from a lesion of the left supramarginal and angular gyri, but there is controversy as to whether this is a distinct entity or merely represents one of a variety of combined defects resulting from lesions of the parietal cortex. Unilateral spatial agnosia and prosopagnosia are usually due to a parieto-occipital lesion of the non-dominant hemisphere. In other types of agnosia the lesions are usually extensive and may be bilateral but we cannot say that there is an exact anatomical localisation for each type of agnosia.

Further Reading

CRITCHLEY M. (1953) *The Parietal Lobes*. Arnold, London.
GESCHWIND N. & BEHAN P. (1982) Left-handedness: association with Immune disease, migraine and developmental learning disorder. *Proc. Natl. Acad. Sci. USA* 79, 5097–100.
NATHAN P.W. (1947) Facial apraxia and apraxic dysarthria. *Brain* 70, 449.

CHAPTER 4
CEREBRAL DOMINANCE

As human behaviour in evolution has become more complex, specialisation of cerebral function has been accentuated and the bilateral symmetry of the brain has been modified both structurally and functionally. Although superficially the paired cerebral hemispheres appear identical, one of them—in man—develops a specialised area which controls language and this is called the dominant hemisphere. For reasons which are not known, the dominant cerebral hemisphere is nearly always the left, and detailed studies have shown structural differences between the left and right temporal gyri. The region between the primary auditory cortex and Wernicke's association area for speech is recognisably larger on the left in most fetuses from the 20th week of intrauterine life, and in adults the left temporoparietal lobe controlling speech, spatial orientation and praxis is slightly larger and contains more nerve cells than the corresponding part of the right hemisphere. Furthermore, the electroencephalogram (see page 130) often shows a lower voltage alpha rhythm over the left hemisphere, and during speech there is a greater increase in blood flow in Broca's area in the left hemisphere than in the corresponding area on the right. Nevertheless, there is some evidence that the non-dominant right hemisphere may also possess some limited language capacity in right-handed adults, being concerned more with verbal comprehension than with verbal expression.

The concept of cerebral dominance is closely related to the problems of aphasia, and as long ago as 1865 Bouillard suggested that cerebral dominance for speech and handedness were in some way interconnected. It was then thought that the laterality of cerebral dominance for language was associated with handedness—i.e. that the left cerebral hemisphere was dominant for speech in right-handers and the right hemisphere in left-handers. Penfield and Roberts (1959) concluded from studies of cortical stimulation and excision in patients with epilepsy that the left cerebral hemisphere was dominant for speech in nearly everyone, whether left-handed or right-handed, provided that one excluded cases of pathological left-handedness (i.e. due to trauma or disease of the left hemisphere at birth or during infancy).

The present position regarding the relationship between cerebral dominance and handedness is that the left cerebral hemisphere is almost always dominant for speech in right-handers. Examples of right-handers with right cerebral dominance for language are extremely rare, and although this may sometimes be accounted for by damage to the left cerebral hemisphere during development of the brain or at birth, evidence for this is not found in all such cases.

Right-handedness is a feature of the majority of people in all nations and such evidence as is available (e.g. from prehistoric cave paintings and the Bible), suggests that this has always been so. It is not known for certain whether dextrality is an organic or cultural heritage — even the accepted familial trend of sinistrality is unhelpful since this could be either genetic or environmental (or both). An infant does not show any preference for either hand until the age of about 9 months when speech begins. Handedness slowly becomes established with speech — after the age of two, and is undoubtedly governed in some cases by dysgenesis or damage of one cerebral hemisphere. It is now generally recognised that there are varying degrees of laterality, some people being more strongly right-handed than others. True ambidexterity (i.e. the ability to use either hand equally well) is probably quite rare.

Laterality (or sidedness) implies that one side is preferred for certain skills, for example using the hand, foot, eye or ear. Usually there is consistence in the side preferred for a particular skill but laterality depends upon the skill tested, e.g. a person may write with the right hand and throw a ball with the left, yet prefer to kick a ball with the right foot; this is called mixed laterality or mixed dominance. Although there may be a preferred eye (e.g. for looking through a telescope or kaleidoscope), this cannot be related directly to cerebral dominance since the nerve fibres from each eye go to both hemispheres. In any case the eye used may also depend upon which hand is preferred for holding the telescope. Most right-handers appear to have right ear preference (consistent with contralateral hemisphere lateralisation of language), but this may depend largely on which hand is used (e.g. when holding the telephone). Ear advantage has also been tested by dichotic listening; this has shown that only 80% of right-handers have right ear advantage and so the relationship with cerebral dominance (i.e. hemisphere language laterality) is not clear.

Left-handedness

Left-handed subjects are those who prefer to use the left hand for the performance of the majority of one-handed motor skills (e.g. throwing a ball and using a racquet); this may include preference for kicking a ball with the left foot. The prevalence of left-handedness in the general population ranges from 5 to 10%.

Individual variation in the degree of laterality is common among left-handers, and many use their right hand more often and more skilfully than right-handers use their left.

Various methods have been used to try and assess the degree of laterality (e.g. the Oldfield (1971) handedness questionnaire and also noting ear preference and ear advantage in dichotic listening). But none of these methods has proved reliable; neither the degree of sinistrality, nor family history of sinistrality, is a reliable indicator of right hemisphere dominance for language. For example, it might be thought that left-handers who write with the left hand are more strongly left-handed than left-handers who write with the right hand and that they would be more likely to have the right hemisphere dominant; but whether a left-hander uses his left or right hand for writing does not necessarily indicate which hemisphere is dominant, e.g. some left-handers who write with the left hand are rendered aphasic from left hemisphere lesions, and others, also left-handed writers, are rendered aphasic from right hemisphere lesions; the same applies to left-handers who write with the right hand (see page 45). It has also been thought that a normal hand position when writing indicates contralateral language specialisation, but recent studies of transient dysphasia induced by unilateral ECT have not confirmed this (Pratt and Warrington 1972; Warrington and Pratt 1973). These studies have also shown that ear advantage tested by dichotic listening seems to be related to factors such as spatial attention rather than to hemisphere language laterality.

Cerebral dominance for language in left-handers

Definite evidence indicating which cerebral hemisphere is dominant for language is usually only established when a single unilateral cerebral lesion produces dysphasia. Confirmation that the majority of left-handers have left cerebral dominance for language has been obtained, for example, from the study of aphasia due to brain wounds (Russell and Espir 1961). However, the pattern of cerebral dominance for language function in left-handers is complex. It is now clear that the left cerebral hemisphere is dominant for language in about 70% of left-handers. In the remainder, the right cerebral hemisphere may be dominant, though in some both hemispheres may contribute to language function without definite dominance on one side; this is the concept of *cerebral ambilaterality* suggested by Zangwill (1960). Although in some cases of right cerebral dominance there is evidence of trauma or disease of the left hemisphere at birth or during infancy (causing pathological left-handedness), evidence of this is by no means always apparent.

In some cases (e.g. when planning a surgical procedure such as temporal lobectomy for epilepsy) it is important to try and determine preoperatively with as much certainty as possible which cerebral hemisphere is dominant for language, as obviously there is a greater risk of dysphasia developing as a complication from an operation on the dominant hemisphere. Two tests give unequivocal evidence:
1   The intracarotid artery injection of sodium amytal—the Wada test (Milner, Branch and Rasmussen 1964) and
2   Unilateral ECT (Pratt and Warrington 1972). Both these techniques produce transient dysphasia when given on the side of the dominant cerebral hemisphere but not of the non-dominant. Unfortunately both methods are 'invasive' and therefore can only be justified if the information about language laterality (a) cannot be obtained reliably by non-invasive methods and (b) is essential for management (e.g. to help with the assessment of potential risks of neurosurgical treatment). At operation, direct electrical stimulation of the appropriate area of cerebral cortex will confirm whether or not the exposed hemisphere is dominant, but the need remains for a reliable safe non-invasive method of establishing cerebral hemisphere language laterality.

As the left cerebral hemisphere is dominant for language in over 99% of right-handers and at least 70% of left-handers, dysphasia will only rarely result from right hemisphere lesions, but when it does, the patient is likely to be left-handed. It is therefore worth enquiring about handedness, bearing in mind the possibility of dominance of the right cerebral hemisphere or of cerebral ambilaterality. After a lesion of the language area of the dominant cerebral hemisphere, recovery of language may be dependent on the integrity of the non-dominant hemisphere and its capacity to take over language function. This may be possible in early childhood but becomes less likely with increasing age.

References

BOUILLARD J. (1865) *Discussion sur la Faculté du Langage Articule. Bull. Acad. Med. (Paris)* 30, 575.

MILNER B., BRANCH C. & RASMUSSEN T. (1964) *Disorders of Language*, CIBA Foundation Symposium, page 200, ed. by A.V.S. de Reuck and M. O'Connor. Churchill Livingstone, Edinburgh.

OLDFIELD R.C. (1971) The Assessment and Analysis of Handedness: The Edinburgh Inventory. *Neuropsychologia* 91, 97–113.

PENFIELD W. & ROBERTS L. (1959) *Speech and Brain Mechanisms.* University Press, Princeton.

PRATT R.T.C. & WARRINGTON E.K. (1972) The Assessment of Cerebral Dominance with Unilateral ECT. *Brit. J. Psychiat.* 121, 327–8.

RUSSELL W.R. & ESPIR M.L.E. (1961) *Traumatic Aphasia.* University Press, Oxford.

WARRINGTON E.K. & PRATT R.T.C. (1973) Language Laterality in Lefthanders. Assessed by Unilateral ECT. *Neuropsychologia* 11, 423–8.

ZANGWILL O.L. (1960) *Cerebral Dominance and Its Relation to Psychological Function.* Oliver and Boyd, Edinburgh.

Further Reading

BENTON A.L. (ed.) (1969) *Contributions to Clinical Neuropsychology.* Aldine Publishing, Chicago.

BISHOP D.V.M. (1980) Handedness, clumsiness and cognitive ability. *Dev. Med. Child. Neurol.* 22, 569–79.

FREEDMAN B.J. (1981) Left and Right. *Brit. Med. J.* 282, 378–9.

GALABURDA A.M. & EIDELBERG D. (1982) Symmetry and Asymmetry in the Human Posterior Thalamus. ii. Thalamic Lesions in a case of Developmental Dyslexia. *Arch. Neurol.* 39, 333–6.

GALABURDA A.M. & KEMPER T.L. (1979) Cytoarchitectonic abnormality in developmental dyslexia: a case study. *Ann. Neurol.* 6, 94–100.

GAZZANIGA M. & HILLYARD S.A. (1971) Language and Speech Capacity of the Right
  Hemisphere. *Neuropsychologia* 9, 273–80.
GEFFEN G., TRAUB E. & STIERMAN I. (1978) Language Laterality Assessed by Uni-
  lateral ECT and Dichotic Monitoring. *J. Neurol. Neurosurg. Psychiat.* **41**,
  354–60.
LEVY J. & REID M. (1976) Variations in Writing Posture and Cerebral Organisation.
  Science **194**, 337–9.
MORAIS J. (1978) Spatial Constraints on Attention to Speech. In *Attention Perform-
  ance*, Vol. 7; ed. by J. Requin.
ROSE F.C. (1965) *8th International Congress of Neurology; Proceedings.* Excerpta
  Medica, Amsterdam.
WADA J. & RASMUSSEN T. (1860) Intracarotid injection of sodium amytal for the
  lateralisation of cerebral speech dominance; experimental and clinical observa-
  tion. *J. Neurosurg.* **17**, 266–82.
WYKE M. (1971) Dysphasia: A Review of Recent Progress. *Brit. Med. Bull* **27**, 3,
  211–17.
ZANGWILL O.L. (1967) Speech and the Minor Hemisphere. *Acta. Neurol. Belg.* **67**,
  1013–20.

CHAPTER 5
DYSPHASIA

History

Probably the earliest case of aphasia ever recorded is in the first chapter of the Gospel according to St Luke, where Zacharias was struck dumb but could still write (vv 20–22, and 62–64), and the next in Roman times, when about AD 30 Valerius Maximus described a learned man of Athens who lost his memory for letters after being struck by a stone. There were several reports of aphasia in the seventeenth, and eighteenth centuries by Linnaeus the great botanist, Morgagni, Heberden and also Goethe in his novel *Wilhelm Meister*.

The early descriptions explained aphasia on a motor basis in terms of paralysis of the tongue and other organs of speech ('The dead palsy'), and occasionally as part of a general loss of mental faculties (Willis 1683). A century later, when it was observed that aphasia could occur without motor paralysis and without overall dementia, the phenomenon was classed as a defect of memory. With the influence of phrenological studies in the nineteenth century, specific cerebral lesions of the organ of language were described.

In April 1861 Dr Paul Broca had under his care at the Bicêtre Hospital in Paris a speechless hemiplegic patient. The patient eventually died and, at post-mortem examination, a cavity the size of a hen's egg was found in the posterior third of the left second and third frontal convolutions (the equivalent of Brodmann's area 44). This was demonstrated by Broca at a meeting of the *Société d'Anthropologie de Paris*; and as similar cases were collected, he formed the axiom: *on parle avec l'hémisphère gauche*. (There is controversy as to whether the priority given to Broca for his discovery is justified. Dr Mark Dax of Montpellier, according to his son Gustave, had written a paper in 1836 to the effect that lesions interfering with speech lay in the left hemisphere. This paper was not published until 1865 and Broca did not know about it at the

29

time of his original communication.) Broca called the speech disorder 'aphemia'; previously it had been called 'alalia'. The term aphasia, which had been used in a philosophical sense in the second century AD by the Romans, was reintroduced by Trousseau in 1864. Following this, the concept of cerebral dominance was developed (see Chapter 4).

During the last 100 years there has been considerable debate as to the best way in which to classify the disorders of speech which result from a lesion of the dominant cerebral hemisphere, and writers on the subject have included Hughlings Jackson, Head, Brain and Critchley in this country, Marie and Déjerine in France, Henschen and Kleist in Germany, Luria in Russia, and Benson and Geschwind in the United States.

As mentioned in Chapter 2, there is still controversy as to whether various parts of the cortex are solely concerned with specific functions and whether a lesion of part of the speech mechanism will produce some impairment of all its aspects. Pierre Marie in 1906 attacked the existing theories regarding aphasia (and for this reason was described by Head as 'the iconoclast') and later in 1917, with his colleague Foix, demonstrated the anatomical extent of the speech territory from a study of brain wounds, identifying five zones, lesions of which produced particular varieties of speech disorders. They concluded that pure motor aphasia ('anarthrie') was the only speech disorder that could occur in isolation. In 1926 Head reported a series of 26 cases and his work achieved great significance from the fine detail in which his patients were studied and the brilliant discussion of the problems revealed by the clinical findings. Kleist (1934) reported detailed studies of similar material from Germany but, unlike Head, he attempted to elucidate a large number of clinical syndromes, each corresponding with small areas of cortical damage. Henschen (1920, 1922) also attempted to localise separate aspects of language function with evidence from over 1300 cases in the literature.

Whereas before and during the early part of the twentieth century, most workers concentrated on localisation of speech functions and tended to ignore their setting in the hierarchy of higher cerebral function, the pendulum has swung back again to the holistic approach linking speech with memory and the other mental faculties.

Meaningful speech is associated with the ability to think, formulate propositions, choose words and construct sentences. The faculty of language also includes the ability to understand, remember and repeat spoken words, and to read and write. The pathophysiology of aphasia is the most difficult in neurology.

Definition

Aphasia may be defined as loss of the ability to formulate, express or understand the meaning of spoken words, due to a lesion of the language area of the dominant cerebral hemisphere. In addition there may be difficulty in reading (dyslexia), in writing (dysgraphia) and failure to understand gestures, signs (asymbolia) or music (amusia). Aphasia is thus a linguistic disorder with disruption of expression, fluency and/or comprehension of spoken language, sometimes with impairment of the ability to repeat words or sentences, and is due to a focal cerebral lesion. It has to be distinguished from general mental confusion and dementia which result from more diffuse cerebral disorders causing disturbances of thought processes, intellectual ability and behaviour as well as memory and language function.

The terms aphasia, alexia, etc, strictly indicate a complete loss of function, whereas dysphasia, dyslexia, etc, imply partial loss; however, the prefixes a- and dys- are often used interchangeably. They are also commonly applied to childhood disorders of development of language (e.g. developmental dysphasia) although strictly defined, dysphasia is a disorder of language already acquired, and there are differences between this and the deficits due to delayed and disordered development of language (see Chapter 9) —differences in the types of defect as well as in their mechanisms of production.

Clinical types

Traditionally dysphasia has been classified as (a) *motor or expressive* when there is difficulty speaking, resulting from a lesion of Broca's area (i.e. in the posterior part of the inferior frontal convolution) and (b) *sensory or receptive* when there is difficulty understanding, resulting from a lesion of Wernicke's area (i.e. in the posterior part of the superior temporal gyrus). Although either expressive or receptive defects may predominate, usually there are elements of both, often combined with difficulty in writing (dysgraphia) and in reading (dyslexia). Disruption of all aspects of language has been called *global* or *central aphasia*. This classification is now regarded as inadequate and has been superseded by the description of dysphasic disorders as 'non-fluent' or 'fluent' (see Table 1).

Table 1   Distinguishing features of main forms of aphasia.

Type of aphasia	Fluency	Repetition	Comprehension
Broca's	Non-fluent	↓	+
Transcortical motor	Non-fluent	+	+
Wernicke's	Fluent	↓	↓
Transcortical sensory	Fluent	+	↓
Conduction	Fluent	↓	+

+ relatively intact
↓ impaired

Non-fluent dysphasia

There is defective formation of words and when severe the patient may be unable to talk spontaneously. The difficulty with expression interferes with the construction of sentences, patients producing fewer words in short phrases and sentences. They also tend to speak slowly with disturbances of inflection, accent and rhythm (*dysprosody*) and may articulate poorly (*dysarthria*). They commonly realise their disability and are disinclined to attempt to speak, so aggravating their non-fluency.

In less severe cases, or during recovery, the patient may speak in a telegram style leaving out prepositions and conjunctions (*telegrammatism*) with a general poverty of spontaneous speech. There may be grammatical errors (*paragrammatism* or *syntactical aphasia*) with confusion of articles and conjunctions. Disorders of word formation sometimes cause spoonerisms, use of wrong words and difficulty with word-finding. *Perseveration* of words is also a characteristic feature; it is the inappropriate repetition of the same words or phrases in reply to different questions. Patients with non-fluent dysphasia usually understand conversation though not always perfectly, as evidenced by failure with commands such as 'when I lift up my hand, touch your nose'. Loss of fluency with conversational speech, impaired ability to repeat spoken language and difficulty in finding words and names but relatively normal comprehension is called *Broca's aphasia*. The causative lesion is in Broca's area; if it also involves the adjacent motor cortex, it will cause a contralateral hemiparesis affecting particularly the lower part of the face and hand.

Fluent dysphasia

Patients speak more rapidly than normal using more words and phrases (*logorrhoea*) but with normal rhythm and articulation. Wrong words or sounds (*verbal or literal paraphasia*) and neo-logisms result in meaningless or unintelligible speech (*jargon*). Words although heard are not understood, or they fail to convey their normal meaning. In less severe cases, individual words may be recognised and understood but the meaning of sentences is not appreciated. This could be classified as an agnosia for words and has been called auditory-word deafness.

The use of the term 'deafness' in this context is not due to any defect of the peripheral mechanism of hearing, but to a failure to appreciate the significance or meaning of sounds transmitted to, or received by, the auditory area. Destruction of the auditory areas bilaterally causes 'cortical deafness' (i.e. a complete failure to recognise any sound even though the peripheral mechanism for hearing is intact).

Fluent dysphasia with failure to understand and to repeat spoken language is called *Wernicke's aphasia* and is due to a lesion in Wernicke's area. If this extends deeply to involve the optic radia-tion, it will cause a contralateral homonymous hemianopia. In other cases, fluent aphasia is associated with normal comprehen-sion but failure to repeat words correctly. This is *conduction aphasia*, and these patients are unable to read aloud or write and usually have some apraxia. The lesion lies deep in the parietal lobe just above the Sylvian fissure involving the arcuate fasciculus in the supramarginal gyrus, i.e. in the pathway joining Broca's and Wernicke's areas (see Fig. 5).

The lesions involving the perisylvian area invariably interfere with the ability to repeat spoken language. A rare type of aphasia occurs in which patients can repeat what is said but speak very little or not at all spontaneously (transcortical motor aphasia), and/or

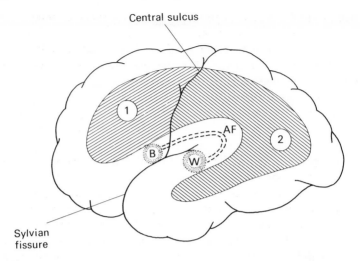

Fig. 5 Anatomical areas involved in main forms of aphasia. (Redrawn from *Aphasia, Alexia and Agraphia* by D.F. Benson, 1979). B = Broca's area; W = Wernicke's area; AF = Arcuate Fasciculus; 1 = Area involved in transcortical motor aphasia; 2 = Area involved in transcortical sensory aphasia.

cannot understand (transcortical sensory aphasia) due to involvement of the association cortex of the frontal and/or parietal lobes, sparing the perisylvian region. This may result from carbon monoxide poinsoning or anoxia.

Global aphasia

Global aphasia is due to lesions of the entire perisylvian region so that there is inability to speak, comprehend or repeat; reading, writing or making gestures are also impaired, usually with apraxias.

Anomic or nominal aphasia

Anomic or nominal aphasia (difficulty in naming and word finding) is not of specific localising value. It may be associated with diffuse as well as focal cerebral lesions. Some patients are unaware of their mistakes but those with nominal aphasia will usually recognise the correct name when it is offered. This could be due to a loss of memory for the appropriate word (amnestic aphasia). There may also be a failure to recognise the significance or intention of words or phrases (*semantic aphasia*).

Dysphasia, in addition to causing difficulty in speaking, often affects the intellect as well but the patient retains *non-propositional speech*. This consists of:

1 *Emotional utterances:*
(a) ejaculations or expostulations
(b) 'Yes' and 'No' which are primitive words in the sense that they are among the first to be learnt
(c) other words used inappropriately or without regard to their proper sense
(d) *jargon*, where words are meaningless and unintelligible
(e) *recurrent utterances* of words or phrases which are sometimes those that were used just before the lesion occurred.
2 *Automatic speech:* such as songs and poems.
3 *Serial speech:* such as the alphabet, days of the week or months of the year.
4 *Social gesture speech:* such as 'How do you do' or 'Goodbye'.

Some of these forms of speech may be retained by virtue of the contribution of the non-dominant hemisphere.

EXAMINATION OF THE APHASIC PATIENT

There are numerous formal tests of language function and many different methods of clinical and psychological assessment of aphasia (e.g. Schuell's, Boston, etc) some differing only in detail and in order of tests performed. Very often the difficulty will be obvious when talking to the patient, but this is not always the case and, in some patients, deficits are only detectable with structured tests. Detailed analysis is time-consuming and is usually undertaken by the specialists directly concerned with the management of language problems, the aphasiologist and speech therapist.

For routine clinical purposes, a brief evaluation under the following headings, based on the Boston programme, is helpful in distinguishing the main aphasic syndromes and localising the causative lesion. Assessment is made of spontaneous speech, comprehension of spoken language, repetition, naming and word finding, reading, writing, praxis and drawing ability. In addition, the language and educational background of the patient is obviously

important, and details of the patient's general mental state, ability
to attend, cooperate and memorise should also be noted.

It is important to remember that a dysphasic patient fatigues
more easily than the normal person and that concentration is
impaired. For these reasons several interviewing periods may be
necessary, particularly to examine the many aspects which may be
relevant, as outlined below. Many dysphasia patients will also
have a homonymous hemianopia, usually on the right, and they
should be approached and spoken to from their seeing side.

Clinical assessment

1   Preliminary assessment of:
    (a) general mental state, e.g. disorientation in space and time,
    confusion
    (b) hearing
    (c) vision, e.g. homonymous hemianopia or other visual field
    defect
    (d) motor function, e.g. hemiparesis.
2   Cerebral dominance: which hand, leg or eye is preferred.
3   Receptive function:
    (a) response to spoken questions and commands, initially
    simple and then more complex
    If incorrect response, note whether mistakes are recognised.
    (b) response to written questions and commands, picking out
    from a group of objects the one that is written down.
4   Expressive function:
    (a) speech—spontaneity, quantity and fluency
    The correctness of word formation, sentence construction and
    reading
    The presence of emotional speech, the lack of propositional
    speech
    Singing better than speech
    Repetition of words and sentences
    Serial speech, e.g. letters of the alphabet, days of the week,
    months of the year, well-known sayings
    In polyglot patients ascertain which languages have been lost
    Naming objects if nominal defect; can use of objects be
    described
    Recognition of correct names and colours

(b) writing—spontaneous (not only name and address, which are often 'automatic') names of objects shown, writing to dictation, copy writing
(c) spelling.
5   Other symbolic functions:
Reading numbers aloud
Writing numbers to dictation
Copying numbers, or copying numbers written as digits and numbers as words
Copying geometric figures
Drawing
Calculation
Music.
6   Apraxia:
Use of objects (e.g. matches, comb, scissors, eating utensils)
Simple movements (e.g. putting out tongue, showing teeth, waving goodbye, dressing)
Complicated actions.
7   Agnosia and disorders of body image:
Distinction between right and left, getting in and out of bed, finding way, recognition of objects, test for finger agnosia.

CAUSES OF APHASIA

The pathological conditions which most commonly cause aphasia are:
1   Cerebral vascular disorders, including haemorrhage from an aneurysm or angioma (see Chapter 17).
2   Brain injuries (see Chapter 19).
3   Intracranial tumours (see Chapter 18).
4   Cerebral abscess (see Chapter 16).
   In fact there are many diseases which can interfere with the cerebral control of speech and language. Aphasia is thus not a pathological diagnosis, but a manifestation of any lesion of the language area of the dominant cerebral hemisphere. Occasionally it occurs as an isolated deficit, although in most cases there are associated disturbances of cerebral function, such as a right upper motor neurone type of facial weakness or hemiparesis. However,

the aphasia and hemiparesis may develop or recover independently of each other.

Although the location and extent of the lesion determine the type and severity of the aphasia, the mode of onset and course depend on the pathology. As a rule a sudden onset with gradual recovery typifies cerebral infarction. Transient dysphasia can occur as the aura of migraine attacks. Brief recurrent stereotyped disturbances of speech are usually due to transient ischaemic attacks or focal epilepsy. Abrupt onset of dysphasia sometimes following an epileptic attack can occur with an abscess or tumour although the latter usually runs a progressive course.

Language may also be affected in patients with dementia but this is then part of a general impairment of mental faculties due to diffuse cerebral disorders such as Alzheimer's disease (see Chapter 13). Distinguishing dysphasia, in which only language is disturbed, is important as this reflects a focal cerebral lesion which may be amenable to surgical treatment.

Developmental speech and language disorders are described separately (see Chapter 9).

PROGNOSIS OF APHASIA

The degree of recovery from aphasia depends upon many factors. Obviously the first step after analysing the clinical deficit is to diagnose and if possible treat the underlying cause. The advent of the CT scan providing a non-invasive method of localising and diagnosing intracranial lesions has transformed management (see page 161).

In addition to identifying the type and severity of the language disturbance, any associated speech disorder and other neurological deficits (e.g. homonymous hemianopia, hemiplegia, etc) should be taken into consideration. The distinction from dementia is very important, as is the level of language that remains intact, so that it is put to maximum use to compensate for residual difficulties.

Although there is controversy concerning the efficacy of different types of speech therapy, and the chances of long-term benefit may be uncertain, we believe that patients with dysphasia due to a non-progressive cause should be referred to a speech therapist as early as possible. Analysis of the speech disorder, serial assessment of any changes and planning of treatment can then be undertaken. The speech therapist may also be in the best position to advise relatives and friends how they can give optimum assistance and make use of volunteer helpers, stroke clubs and aphasia groups. Everything should be done to counter depression, encourage, stimulate and motivate towards maximum recovery and use of residual language.

The chief factors on which the prognosis may depend are as follows:

1 The site and extent of the lesion (e.g. which part and how much of the speech area has been affected, whether the non-dominant hemisphere and commissures have been damaged).

2 The cause of the lesion (e.g. whether the pathological process is reversible or progressive, benign or malignant).

3 Treatment of the cause, response to drugs or radiotherapy, whether surgical removal of a tumour has been total or partial.

4 Speech therapy, stage when started.

5 The severity and clinical type of dysphasia, the more severe the dysphasia, the greater the amount of recovery required. Severe receptive defects may make it impossible for speech therapy to be given. Associated language defects are also important (e.g. dyslexia and dysgraphia).

6 (a) Associated non-language defects (e.g. impairment of other mental functions, particularly memory). Dementia, confusion and disorientation will limit cooperation, and any apraxia, agnosia or other perceptual disorder will interfere with rehabilitation

(b) Other disabilities may include defects of visual fields (*homonymous hemianopia*), unilateral motor or sensory deficits (*hemiplegia* or *hemianaesthesia*), pseudobulbar palsy, ocular palsies causing double vision (*diplopia*), vertigo and epilepsy.

7 (a) Psychological factors (e.g. inability to concentrate, to cooperate and to adjust to limitations, depression, anxiety, emotional lability)

(b) Environmental factors (e.g. home and social conditions, help from relatives, encouragement and reassurance).

8 Age, the older the patient, the poorer the prognosis.

9 Cerebral dominance (see Chapter 4).

10 Premorbid language and intellectual ability, personality and temperament.

References

BENSON D.F. & GESCHWIND N. (1971) *The Aphasias and Related Distrubances.* In *Clinical Neurology* 1, ed. by A.B. Baker and L.H. Baker. Harper and Row, Hagerstown.

BRAIN W.R. (1965) *Speech Disorders 2e.* Butterworths, London.

BROCA P.P. (1861) Perte de la parole: ramollissement chronique et destruction partielle du lobe anterieur gauche du cerveau. *Bull. Soc. Anthrop. (Paris)*, **21**, 235.

DEJERINE J.L. (1914) *Semiologie des Affections du Systeme Nerveux.* Masson et Cie, Paris.

GESCHWIND N. (1971) Aphasia. *New Eng. J. Med.* **284**, 654–56.

HEAD H. (1926) *Aphasia and Kindred Disorders of Speech.* 2 Vols. University Press, Cambridge.

HENSCHEN S.E. (1920) *Klinische und anatomische Beitrage zur Pathologie des Gehirns.* Part 5, Uber Aphasie, Amusie and Akalkulie. Part 6, Uber sensorische Aphasie. Nordiska Bokhandeln, Stockholm.

JACKSON, J. HUGHLINGS (1932) *Selected Writings,* ed. by J. Taylor. Hodder and Stoughton, London.

KLEIST K. (1934) Kriegsverletzungen des Gehirns in ihrer Bedeutung für die Hirnlokalisation und Hirnpathologie. In *Handbuch der Arztlichen Erfahrungen im Weltkriege 1914/1918* (ed. by O. Schjerning). **4**, *Geistes-und Nervenkrankheiten* (ed. by K. Bonhoeffer), pp. 686–933. Barth, Leipzig.

MARIE P. (1906) Revision de la Question de L'Aphasie; la Troisieme Circonvolution Frontale Gauche ne joue aucun Role Special dans la Fonction du Langage. *Sem. Med. (Paris)*, **26**, 241.

MARIE P. ET FOIX Ch. (1917) Les Aphasies de Guerre. *Revue Neurologique*, **24** (i), 53.

TROUSSEAU A. (1864) De l'aphasie. *Gaz. Hop. (Paris)*, **37**, 13.

WILLIS T. (1683) *Two Discourses Concerning the Soul of Brutes.* Prodage, London.

Further Reading

ALBERT M.L., GOODGLASS H., HELM N.A. *et al* (1981) *Clinical Aspects of Dysphasia.* Springer-Verlag Wien, Berlin.

BENSON D.F. (1979) *Aphasia, Alexia and Agraphia.* Churchill Livingstone, Edinburgh.

BUTLER R.B. & BENSON D.F. (1974) Aphasia: a Clinical-Anatomical Correlation. *Brit. J. Hosp. Med.* **12**, 211–17.

CRITCHLEY M. (1970) *Aphasiology; and Other Aspects of Language.* Arnold, London.

DARLEY F.L. (1972) The efficacy of language rehabilitation in aphasia. *J. Speech Hearing Dis.* **37**, 3–21.

GOODGLASS H. & KAPLAN E. (1972) *The Assessment of Aphasia and Related Disorders.* Lea & Febiger, Philadelphia.

JENKINS J.J., JIMENEZ-PABON E., SHAW R.E. *et al* (1970) *Schuell's Aphasia in Adults; Diagnosis, Prognosis and Treatment*, 2e. Harper and Row, Hagerstown.

KERSCHENSTEINER M., POECK K. & BRUNNER E. (1972) The fluency-non fluency dimension in the classification of aphasic speech. *Cortex* **8**, 233–47.

RIOCH D.M. & WEINSTEIN E.A. (1964) *Disorders of Communication*. Williams and Wilkins, Baltimore.

ROSE F.C., BOBY V. & CAPILDER R. (1976) *A Retrospective Survey of Speech Disorders Following Stroke with Particular Reference to the Value of Speech Therapy*. In *Recovery in Asphasics*, ed. by R. Hoops and Y. Lebrun. Swets & Zeitlinger, Amsterdam.

SARNO M.T. (1981) *Acquired Aphasia*. Academic Press, New York.

WEPMAN J.M. (1951) *Recovery from Aphasia*. Ronald Press, New York.

WEPMAN J.M. (1973) *Rehabilitation and the Language Disorders*. In *Rehabilitation Practices with the Physically Disabled*, ed. by J.F. Garnett and E.S. Levine. Columbia University Press, New York.

CHAPTER 6
DYSLEXIA

In this chapter we are concerned with acquired dyslexia, a disruption of the established ability to read which results from the same pathological conditions involving the dominant cerebral hemisphere as those causing dysphasia (see page 37). Developmental dyslexia in which there is delay or prolonged difficulty in *learning to read* has different implications, particularly with regard to its aetiology and management, and is considered separately (see Chapter 9). Whether or not the patterns of loss of an established faculty help to increase our understanding of the mechanisms required for its development is uncertain.

The ability to read is a highly complex aspect of language in which visual patterns produced by letters, words, numbers and music are both recognised and understood. What is read must also be stored long enough to be correlated with what comes later. The neuronal system concerned with storing the visual symbol patterns or with keeping them available for use lie in substantial regions of the parietal and temporal lobes (cortex and tracts) which overlie the optic radiation in the dominant cerebral hemisphere.

Visual mechanisms of the brain make a major contribution to speech, to the acquisition of vocabulary, and to certain forms of mental activity including memory, thought and learning. The visual contribution to speech organisation is concerned also with visual memory of all kinds, as well as with the capacity for visual learning. The ability to name objects seen is partly a process of recognition which may be disorganised from the visual aspect, although the word may be stored in such a way that it can still be used effectively for spontaneous speech. The understanding of words by sound and their production by speaking are the more fundamental aspects of speech, and they may continue to be relatively effective when reading is difficult or impossible.

When learning to read, the following storage systems must be laid down and then made available for use:

1 Visual patterns for the recognition of letters and words.
2 Associations which add meaning to the words.
3 The capacity to hold something of what is read for long enough to correlate it with later pages.

The fornix-hippocampal system facilitates the storage of current happenings and so the patient who cannot remember the previous pages that he has read might have a lesion either of the hippocampal system or of the storage mechanisms in the posterior parietal lobes.

Dyslexia (difficulty in reading) and dysgraphia (difficulty in writing) are constant features in patients with global aphasia, although some can still read aloud although it has no meaning for them, either because they fail to understand or remember what has been read. The patient who can no longer enjoy reading a book may be able to read slowly but have difficulty absorbing the meaning. If the memory of the previous pages is inadequately stored so that he 'loses the thread' the effort to read intelligently becomes fruitless.

Lesions which cause dyslexia involve the posterior part of the dominant parietal lobe in its lower part (i.e. the region of the angular gyrus), but some lesions are further forward and may involve connections with the thalamus.

Lesions overlying the optic radiation in the posterior parietal region are liable to cause difficulty with reading as a relatively isolated disability; this is not directly due to the visual field defects since a homonymous hemianopia may not be present. These lesions may also cause indistinctness or disorientation in the contralateral homonymous half-fields, and sometimes movement in the intact half-fields suppresses recognition of simultaneous movement in the affected field (visual inattention). These phenomena of altered threshold are produced by lesions removed from the optic radiation and illustrate the variety of influences which must operate on various aspects of visual perception and recognition. Loss of visual memory is also known to result from posterior parietal lobe lesions.

Spelling is naturally connected functionally with reading and writing, and for many people visual imagery is very much involved in correct spelling. Most of those with posterior parietal lesions have difficulties with spelling as well as with reading and writing.

If a unilateral left parietal lobe lesion also destroys the commissural fibres crossing in the posterior part (splenium) of the corpus callosum, the intact right parietal lobe will not be able to cooperate with the dominant left temporal lobe, so interfering with the visual aspects of speech, memory and thought.

Dyslexia occasionally occurs without dysgraphia (and vice versa, see page 45). Inability of a patient to read even what he himself has written fluently and grammatically five minutes beforehand was first described by Déjerine (1892). On the basis of postmortem findings from one case he postulated that the syndrome resulted from damage to the left visual cortex combined with a disconnection of the intact visual cortex in the right hemisphere from the language centres of the left hemisphere. Words, although perceived normally in the left homonymous visual fields using the right occipital cortex, could not be transmitted to the intact speech association areas in the left hemisphere due to the interruption of impulses which would normally cross to the left hemisphere through the splenium of the corpus callosum. Thus, although Dejerine's patient could perceive words adequately in the left homonymous visual field, he was able to interpret them as verbal symbols only by using an alternative sensory pathway like touch; he was thus able to read by tracing out letters with his fingers.

In most cases, dyslexia without dysgraphia has been due to cerebrovascular lesions, and in only a few to a tumour. Three patients have been left-handed, and in one of these the cerebral lesion was on the right.

As already mentioned, not all patients with dyslexia have a right homonymous hemianopia, which shows that the syndrome can exist in the presence of an intact left visual cortex if the association fibres leading from it to the speech area have been interrupted.

DYSGRAPHIA

Dysgraphia or agraphia is a disorder of writing caused by a lesion of the dominant cerebral hemisphere. It is not simply an effect of paralysis of the right hand as it can occur without this. If the hand normally used for writing is paralysed, the disorder of writing can be shown to affect the other hand. Dysgraphia thus refers not to any difficulty holding the pen or pencil, but to a disorder of language or an inability to use written symbols correctly, resulting in mistakes with letter, word or sentence construction, and sometimes wrong words or even jargon are written.

Writing is dependent not only on language but also on spatial matters concerning the writer's hand, the writing surface and the relative shape and position of letters. There are a variety of storage systems in the brain concerned with the shape of letters of the alphabet, numerals, music, etc, and from these comes the ability to connect letters for copying, spelling and expression in writing with the personal characteristics of writing which are so strongly developed in the individual. This storage system requires the integrity of the superior and inferior parietal lobules and the underlying white matter.

The term agraphia was introduced by Ogle (1867), and the literature on the subject was reviewed by Penfield & Roberts (1959). Many, including Wernicke (1874), have postulated a writing centre in the second left frontal gyrus, but Head (1926) rejected this attempt to separate writing from other aspects of speech. Kleist (1934) and Critchley (1953) suggested that agraphia might be a form of apraxia. Dysgraphia with dyslexia usually results from lesions of the angular gyrus, and comes into the category of visual asymbolia. An isolated form of agraphia in which reading is relatively preserved may be due to a lesion of the parasagittal region of the parietal lobe. If the lesion extends deeply to involve the area of the brain concerned with correlations of the body image and spatial orientation, other forms of apraxia and parietal lobe syndromes ensue. Dysgraphia may thus be associated with dyspraxia for other motor skills but not necessarily so. Although dysgraphia may be a dyspraxia for writing, it cannot always be separated from other aspects of language, and dysgraphia is usually a prominent feature of global aphasia. Nevertheless, parasagittal lesions in the posterior part of the left parietal lobe can produce a disorder of writing which is more severe than other dysphasic features, and rarely a relatively pure agraphia can be recognised among the varieties of aphasia.

Handedness is of special importance in relation to writing. Although some left-handed people write with the right hand, very few right-handed people write with the left hand. In right-handers, there is a clear connection between handedness for writing and the dominant hemisphere for speech but, in left-handers, although the left hemisphere is dominant in most, some of them write with the right hand and some with the left, and the effect on writing when a cerebral lesion causes aphasia is of great interest. It used to be thought that left-handers who write with the left hand are more strongly left-handed than left-handers who write with the right hand and so would be more likely to have right hemisphere dominance. In fact, with whichever hand left-handers prefer to write, it does not necessarily indicate which hemisphere is dominant. Thus whether they prefer the left or right hand for writing, the left hemisphere is usually dominant and so, if damaged, dysphasia and dysgraphia can result. A small number of left-handers are rendered dysphasic and dysgraphic from right hemisphere lesions, but this again does not depend on whether they write with their left hand or right hand.

Further Reading

BENSON D.F. (1979) *Aphasia, Alexia and Agraphia.* Churchill Livingstone, Edinburgh.

KIRSHNER H.S. & WEBB W.G. (1982) Alexia and agraphia in Wernicke's aphasia. *J. Neurol. Neurosurg. Psychiat.* **45**, 719–24.

CHAPTER 7
DYSARTHRIA

Dysarthria is defined as disordered articulation of speech, while anarthria is the complete inability to articulate words. Articulation is the process whereby sounds produced by respiratory movements and phonation are converted into the acoustic symbols (words) required for speech. The ability to articulate clearly is dependent in the first place on the normal anatomical arrangement of the mouth, teeth, and nasopharynx. A hot potato in the mouth, of course, disrupts articulation—albeit temporarily—and those with missing front teeth cannot pronounce 't' or 'the' clearly but this is usually correctable. With structural oral deformities, whether congenital (for example cleft palate) or acquired (such as neoplasm of the tongue), the nature of the difficulty varies according to which part of the articulatory apparatus is involved. The terms dysarthria and anarthria are best restricted to defects of articulation, partial and complete respectively, resulting from neuromuscular disorders, where the complex processes that control and coordinate the movements of the lips, tongue, and palate are involved. Stammering is considered separately (see Chapter 10), and the authors do not use the term dysarthria to cover all motor speech disorders.

The initiation, control, and coordination of the movements of the articulatory muscles depend on the normal development and functioning of specific parts of the motor areas of the cerebral hemispheres and on the integrated action of the upper motor neurones, basal ganglia, and cerebellum. The impulses generated are then transmitted to the lower motor neurones in the brainstem, that is the motor nuclei of the 7th, 9th, 10th, 11th, and 12th cranial nerves which innervate the articulatory muscles. The normal development of articulation in the child depends also on sensory input, that is hearing, kinaesthetic sensations, and feedback from the articulatory structures.

The cortical representation of articulation is in the lower part of the posterior frontal region of both cerebral hemispheres. In the dominant hemisphere this is connected directly with Broca's area (the anterior part of the language area) and the corresponding motor part of the nondominant hemisphere is connected with Broca's area via the corpus callosum. Together these regions are concerned with the elaboration of the movement patterns required not only for articulation but also for the laryngeal and respiratory movements which combine to produce normal speech.

Phonation is the production of vocal sounds resulting from the passage of currents of air through the larynx. The strength, tone, pitch, and resonance of the voice are likewise dependent on the structure and neuromuscular control of the laryngeal and respiratory systems. With normal articulation various types of phonemes are pronounced, not only with the action of the articulatory muscles but also with alterations of the airstream. With stop-plosives (p, b, t, d, k, and g) these phonemes are produced by complete stoppage, build-up of pressure, and sudden release. With fricatives (f, v, th, th, s, z, sh, zh, and h) the block is less complete, while with affricates (ch and j) the airstream is constricted. With glides (wh, w, and y) there is hardly any blockage of the airstream, as with semivowels (r and l). The nasal consonants (m, n, and ng) are produced by using the nasal cavity as a resonator and so differ from those where the emission is oral.

Phonemes are thus given their correct form by movements of lips, tongue and palate and any abnormality of this sytem produces defects or difficulty in articulation, hypo- or hypernasality or changes in intonation. Some disorders cause weakness or hoarseness of the voice (*dysphonia*) which may be reduced to just a whisper while articulation remains normal; with other disorders articulation may be defective without dysphonia. Some neuromuscular conditions can affect both articulation and phonation, and the term dysarthrophonia describes this combination.

NEUROLOGICAL CAUSES OF DYSARTHRIA

The neurological causes of dysarthria are classified according to which part of the neuromuscular system is affected. The disorders may thus involve:

1 Muscles.
2 Lower motor neurones.
3 Upper motor neurones.

4 Extrapyramidal system.
5 Cerebellum and its connections.
6 Cerebral cortex (motor speech area).
7 Combinations of the above.
and will be described under these headings.

DISORDERS OF MUSCLES

All our active movements such as breathing, performing manoeuvres with the hands and walking, are dependent upon the action
of muscles. Likewise the muscles concerned with articulation are
essential for the production of normal speech. Muscles form 80%
of the body weight and there are over 200 named ones in the body.
Each muscle consists of bundles of microscopic muscle fibres which
are capable of contracting and relaxing under nervous control
mediated by biochemical means. By virtue of the attachments of
muscles, shortening of the fibres resulting from their contraction
produces movement. Individual muscles are supplied by the cranial
or spinal nerves which form the necessary connections with the
brain stem or spinal cord respectively.

Primary disorders of muscles are referred to as 'myopathies'.
They are characterised by weakness and wasting of the muscles
affected with reduction or loss of associated tendon reflexes. The
electrical reactions of the muscle tested by electromyography
(EMG) are abnormal.

The different diseases have a predilection for certain groups of
muscles and can be recognised by the particular pattern and distribution of the muscles affected. Whether speech is involved will
depend upon the type and extent of the disease. The main diseases
that have to be considered are:
1 The muscular dystrophies.
2 Polymyositis.
3 Myasthenia gravis.
The chief characteristics of these diseases are indicated in Table 2.

Table 2 Disorders of muscles (myopathies).

	Pathology and aetiology	Signs and symptoms General	Speech	Treatment
1 Muscular dystrophies	Various types affecting different groups of muscles. Abnormalities of muscle enzymes, usually hereditary	Weakness and wasting of affected muscles. Slow progression	Slurred speech if articulatory muscles involved	Nil specific
2 Polymyositis	Inflammatory disease of muscles and sometimes skin (dermatomyositis). Usually a collagen disease, 10% associated with cancer	Usually proximal muscles weak, painful and tender	May be slurred and slow	Steroids
3 Myasthenia gravis	Auto-immune disorder affecting neuromuscular transmission. Excessive fatiguability of muscles. 10–15% associated with tumour of thymus (thymoma)	Usually affects eye muscles causing diplopia and ptosis. Dysphagia and generalised weakness may occur	Articulation becomes increasingly indistinct (dysarthria) and the voice weak (dysphonia). Recovery following rest or injection of tensilon or prostigmine	Neostigmine or pyridostigmine Thymectomy Immunosuppressant drugs, e.g. steroids azathioprine Plasma exchange

Myasthenia gravis

This is a rare autoimmune disease of unknown cause. Symptoms are due to a disorder of neuromuscular transmission at the myoneural junction. The contraction of voluntary muscle is normally dependent on the release of acetylcholine from the nerve terminal into the synaptic cleft of the motor end plate of each muscle fibre. Here it reacts with specialised acetylcholine receptors and generates an electrical action potential which builds up to trigger the muscle fibre to contract. The acetylcholine is then rapidly destroyed by the enzyme cholinesterase and the process is repeated for each contraction as required. In myasthenia gravis, some of the acetylcholine receptors are damaged and reduced in number by an antibody (anti-acetylcholine receptor antibody). When there are insufficient receptors, muscle contraction cannot be maintained, and after the initial reaction, the muscle tires, becomes weak and fails to contract. This results in the increased fatiguability which is characteristic of this condition so that the muscles tire sooner than normal and become progressively weaker as they are used, with recovery after a period of rest.

The condition may occur at any age but usually between 20 and 50 years; it is slightly more frequent in females. The commonest mode of presentation in about 80% of cases is with ocular symptoms such as double vision (*diplopia*) and drooping of the upper eyelid (*ptosis*). Not infrequently the voice becomes fainter (*dysphonic*) after talking for some time, speech may become slurred and indistinct (*dysarthric*) and there may be difficulty in swallowing (*dysphagia*). The muscles of mastication (*chewing*) may be affected and the jaw may become so weak that it has to be supported by hand. The symptoms, worse in the evenings and after using the affected muscles, are relieved by rest.

The diagnosis is usually established by giving a test dose of edrophonium (tensilon) intravenously. Within a few seconds this blocks the activity of cholinesterase; acetylcholine is then not destroyed so quickly and muscle power is restored temporarily. This relief lasts for a few minutes only and weakness then returns. Alternatively neostigmine (prostigmine) can be given intramuscularly; it has the same effect after about 15 minutes and acts for about an hour. In many cases treatment with neostigmine tablets taken by mouth is effective.

Although the cause of the autoimmune disorder and the anti-acetylcholine receptor antibody production are not known, there appears to be some connection with the thymus, a gland in the anterior part of the mediastinum. Surgical removal of the thymus (*thymectomy*) leads to improvement or remission in 60–80% of patients. Immunosuppressant treatment with drugs such as steroids (e.g. prednisolone) and azathioprine is also effective, and more recently plasma exchange to remove the anti-acetylcholine receptor antibody has been found to produce striking short-term clinical improvement.

About 15% of patients with myasthenia gravis are found to have a thymoma (tumour of the thymus) which requires surgical removal and, in some cases, radiotherapy.

DISORDERS OF LOWER MOTOR NEURONES

The nervous impulses which control movement are transmitted along the motor pathway extending from the cerebral cortex to the peripheral nerves supplying the muscles (see Fig. 3). The motor nuclei of the cranial nerves with their nerve fibres extending to their neuromuscular junctions (the motor end plates) and from the anterior horn cells in the spinal cord with their fibres forming the spinal nerves and extending to their motor end plates constitute the *lower motor neurones* (LMN).

Each nerve fibre supplies a large number of muscle fibres, the number varying with the type of muscles, e.g. the average limb muscle will have about one nerve fibre supplying 100 muscle fibres, whereas in the external ocular muscles the ratio is approximately 1 : 4. The nerve fibre together with the muscle fibres it supplies is called a 'motor unit'. The nerve cells of the lower motor neurones (i.e. the motor nuclei of the cranial nerves and the anterior horn cells of the spinal cord) are controlled by other parts of the nervous system. Thus the initiation and coordination of muscular action, and the control of tone and posture are the result of impulses from the motor nerve cells in the cerebral cortex (the upper motor neurones) interacting with impulses from the cerebellum and basal ganglia and being transmitted across the synapses to the lower motor neurones (see Fig 6).

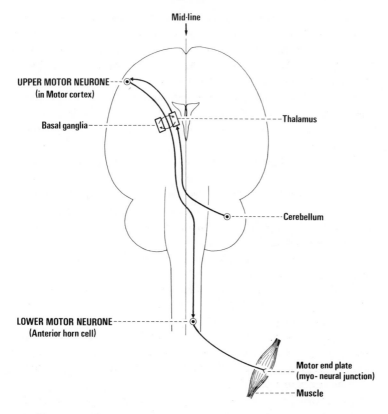

Fig. 6 Diagrammatic representation of control of muscle.

Synapse
A synapse is the gap between the termination of one nerve fibre and the cell body of another neurone, around which there is an area of electrical excitability highly sensitive to the chemical substances responsible for the transmission and modification of impulses.

Disorders of the lower motor neurones are characterised by wasting and weakness of the muscles affected, their tone is decreased leading to flaccidity, and their tendon reflexes are reduced or absent (see Table 5). Electrical studies of nerve conduction and of the affected muscles by electromyography (EMG) show characteristic changes.

In some cases of lower motor neurone involvement, particularly when there is active degeneration of the anterior horn cells, the affected muscles show spontaneous small contractions—fasciculation. This can also be shown on the electromyogram and is a typical feature of motor neurone disease (see Chapter 21).

The lower motor neurones controlling the muscles used for articulation (as well as phonation and swallowing) from the 7th, 9th, 10th, 11th and 12th cranial nerves originate form their motor nuclei in the brain stem. These supply the muscles of the lips, palate, pharynx, larynx and tongue, and knowledge of their anatomy is required.

Seventh cranial (facial) nerve leaves the lower border of the pons on each side and passes through the skull in the facial canal in close proximity to the eighth cranial (acoustic) nerve. It emerges through the stylomastoid foramen and supplies the muscles which control facial expression, movements of the lips, raising the eyebrows, frowning and closing the eyes.

The 9th, 10th and 11th cranial nerves leave the medulla on each side and pass through the skull in the jugular foramen.

Ninth cranial (glossopharyngeal) nerve supplies only one muscle, the stylo-pharyngeus and conveys sensation from the pharynx and posterior third of the tongue including taste.

Tenth cranial (vagus) nerve is formed by several roots emerging from the medulla oblongata. They join to form the intracranial trunk of the vagus nerve which on each side passes through the skull in the jugular foramen. Here the nerve enlarges (ganglion jugulare) to connect with the 7th, 9th, 11th and 12th cranial nerves and sympathetic fibres. After passing through the jugular foramen, the vagus forms another ganglion (ganglion nodosa) which connects with sensory and parasympathetic fibres. Inferior to this ganglion, the pharyngeal plexus is formed by the pharyngeal branches of the vagus, the pharyngeal branches of the glosso-pharyngeal and sympathetic fibres. It is this plexus which innervates the palate and pharynx both sensory and motor, supplying (a) the muscles of the palate (with the exception of the tensor palati which is supplied by the mandibular branch of the 5th nerve) and (b) the muscles of the pharynx, namely the three constrictors, and the salpingo- and palato-pharyngeus, and the stylopharyngeus muscle (see above).

Next to arise from the vagus, below the pharyngeal plexus, is the superior laryngeal nerve. This divides into the internal branch conveying sensation from the laryngeal mucosa above the vocal cords, and the external branch which innervates the cricothyroid muscle. The remaining intrinsic muscles of the larynx are supplied by the recurrent laryngeal nerves which also arise from the vagus but then take a different course on the two sides, on the left curving below the arch of the aorta, and on the right below the subclavian artery. The vagus then descends through the thorax forming cardiac and gastric plexuses and supplying motor, secretory and sensory fibres to the various viscera.

Eleventh cranial (accessory) nerve is a purely motor nerve, composed of two parts, cranial and spinal. The *cranial part* joins the vagus nerve and contributes to the functions described above. The *spinal part* arises from grey matter in the lateral part of the anterior horn of the upper 5 cervical cord segments, and forms a trunk which passes upwards through the foramen magnum; it briefly makes contact with the cranial part of the accessory nerve and the vagus, and with them passes out of the skull again through the jugular foramen. It then supplies the sterno-mastoid and trapezius muscles.

Twelfth cranial (hypoglossal) nerve leaves the lower part of the medulla on each side and passes through the skull in the hypoglossal foramen. It traverses the deep structures of the neck and supplies the muscles of the tongue.

Disorders of lower motor neurones causing dysarthria are divided into two groups, depending on whether there is involvement of the cranial nerves (7th, 9th, 10th, 11th or 12th) or of their motor nuclei in the brain stem.

1 *Disorders of cranial nerves* (7, 9, 10, 11 and 12)
    (a) polyneuritis
    (b) damage by neoplasm, goitre, aneurysm or trauma
    (c) Bell's palsy.
2 *Disorders of motor nuclei in the brain stem*
    (a) poliomyelitis
    (b) motor neurone disease (progressive bulbar palsy)
    (c) syringobulbia
    (d) neoplasm.

For further details of these conditions, see Tables 3 and 4. Dysarthria due to the disorders of the lower motor neurones may form part of the clinical syndrome of bulbar palsy.

Table 3 Disorders of lower motor neurones, involving cranial nerves 7th, 9th, 10th, 11th, 12th.

	Pathology and aetiology	Signs and symptoms		Treatment
		General	Speech	
1 Polyneuritis	Acute type following infections, occasionally glandular fever etc. Chronic cases (e.g. due to diabetes and alcohol)	Symmetrical weakness and sensory changes usually starting in distal parts of limbs and 'muzzle' area of face. Spinal and cranial nerves may be affected	Dysarthria, nasal voice and dysphonia result if the lower cranial nerves are affected due to paresis of lips, palate, pharynx, larynx and tongue	Rest in acute stage, postural drainage or tracheostomy and assisted respiration may be necessary
2 Damage to cranial nerves	Neoplasm Goitre Aneurysm of aorta Trauma	Local effects dependent on the type and site of the pathological lesion	As above	Sometimes surgical
3 Bell's palsy	Inflammatory or ischaemic lesion of 7th cranial (facial) nerve in stylomastoid canal. Usually recovers	Paralysis of the facial muscles on the affected side	Slurred speech due to unilateral facial weakness affecting muscles around the mouth	Physiotherapy for facial muscles. Occasionally steroids or surgery

Table 4 Disorders of lower motor neurones, involving motor nuclei of brain stem.

	Pathology and aetiology	Signs and symptoms		Treatment
		General	Speech	
1 Poliomyelitis	Virus infection of motor nuclei of cranial nerves in brain stem and anterior horn cells of spinal cord. Mild cases are reversible, severe irreversible (see pages 155 and 156)	Paresis or paralysis of limb muscles with wasting and LMN signs. No sensory loss. Bulbar palsy. Respiratory paralysis	Dysarthria Dysphonia	As for polyneuritis
2 Motor neurone disease	Cause unknown. Onset usually in middle age. Progressive deterioration with death usually in 2–4 years (see Chapter 21)	Progressive bulbar palsy. Wasting and fasciculation of tongue, and muscles of limbs (amyotrophy). Pharyngeal weakness with dysphagia. UMNs also involved (see Table 6)	Dysarthria, articulation becomes more indistinct, labials most noticeably affected due to paresis of lips, progressive weakness of tongue impairs dental and velar sounds. Dysphonia, weakness of soft palate causes nasal tone	Nil specific

Table 4—*continued*

	Pathology and aetiology	Signs and symptoms		Treatment
		General	Speech	
3 Syringobulbia (syringomyelia)	Cystic degeneration starting around 4th ventricle and central canal of spinal cord. Developmental disorder. Onset of symptoms usually between 20 and 40. Slowly progressive	Nystagmus. Sensory loss on face associated with manifestations of syringomyelia (i.e. wasting of small muscles of the hands, trophic changes etc)	As above	Surgical decompression occasionally indicated
4 Neoplasm	Glioma—rare in brain stem, usually children (see pages 170 and 176).	Signs of progressive involvement of cranial nerve nuclei, often starting in the pons, may be asymmetrical.	As above	Radiotherapy

BULBAR PALSY

Mechanism of production

Bulbar palsy implies that there is weakness of the muscles supplied by the cranial nerves whose motor nuclei lie in the medulla or bulb. The diseases causing bulbar palsy involve either these motor nuclei, the cranial nerves themselves, their motor end plates or the muscles supplied (see Tables 2, 3 and 4).

Clinical features

The main clinical features are dysarthria, dysphonia and dysphagia due to weakness and wasting of the muscles supplied by the lower cranial nerves. If there is weakness of the jaw muscles, chewing is difficult, the lower jaw droops and there may be dribbling of saliva. Involvement of the facial muscles, particularly the orbicularis oris, affects the bilabial plosives (b and p) and the phonemes requiring lip rounding and spreading; the patient also has difficulty in whistling. With weakness of elevation of the soft palate, the nasopharynx is not closed off properly and there is a nasal sound to the voice (hypernasality or hyperrhinolalia) due to the nasal escape of air, and there may be nasal reflux of fluids when swallowing. The tongue is wasted and flaccid, and in the progressive bulbar palsy due to motor neurone disease, fasciculation in the tongue and other muscles is a characteristic feature.

The dysarthria of bulbar palsy in which the weakness of the muscles is associated with wasting usually affects all consonants and differs from that of pseudobulbar palsy in which the muscle weakness is associated with spasticity.

Associated signs

There may be more generalised lower motor neurone involvement affecting the muscles of the trunk and limbs, supplied by the spinal nerves originating from the affected anterior horn cells of the spinal cord. These muscles will then also develop weakness, wasting and flaccidity with diminution or absence of tendon reflexes.

DISORDERS OF UPPER MOTOR NEURONES

Disorders may affect any part of the upper motor neurone from its cell body in the motor cortex to its termination in the synapse with its appropriate lower motor neurone (Fig. 3). The muscles affected become weak or paralysed with no wasting or just a little due to disuse. The tone of the affected muscles is increased, leading to spasticity which is usually accompanied by the phenomenon of clonus. Clonus is typically elicited by the stimulus of stretching a muscle or group of muscles and consists of the repetitive alternating contraction and relaxation of these muscles. The clonus in severe cases is sustained as long as the stretch stimulus is applied, and can occur spontaneously. The tendon reflexes on the affected side are exaggerated and the plantar response becomes extensor (Babinski's sign). Paralysis may involve one limb (monoplegia), one half of the body (hemiplegia), both legs (paraplegia) or all four limbs (quadriplegia), depending on which of the upper motor neurone fibres are involved.

The main differences between the clinical signs of upper and lower motor neurone lesions are summarised in Table 5.

Table 5   Summary of the differences between upper and lower neurone lesions.

	UMN	LMN
Distribution of weakness	Whole limb or part	Single muscles or groups of muscles
Tone	Increased (spasticity)	Decreased (flaccidity)
Clonus	Present	Absent
Tendon reflexes	Increased	Decreased or absent
Plantar response	Extensor	Flexor or absent
Wasting	Absent	Present
Fasciculation	Absent	Present in some

Most of the motor nuclei of the cranial nerves in the brain stem have bilateral UMN representation. This means that each of these motor nuclei is controlled (a) by corticobulbar fibres which have originated from the contralateral cerebral hemisphere and crossed in the brain stem, i.e. the majority, and (b) by a smaller number of uncrossed corticobulbar fibres which have originated from the ipsilateral cerebral hemisphere. Thus corticobulbar fibres from both cerebral hemispheres (the majority crossed but some uncrossed) form synapses with the motor nuclei on each side of the brain stem. Part of the motor nucleus of the facial nerve supplying the muscles of the *lower* part of the face does not have bilateral representation (i.e. it is controlled only by the crossed corticobulbar fibres originating from the face area of the opposite cerebral hemisphere). If these upper motor neurones are damaged, there will be weakness of the muscles in the lower part of the face on the opposite side; this is in contrast to the *upper* part of the face in which power of the muscles is largely maintained because they are controlled by a different part of the nucleus of the facial nerve which does have bilateral representation, function being preserved by the uncrossed fibres originating from the unaffected cerebral hemisphere. In these cases the weakness of the face is more obvious with emotional movements than with voluntary movements of the facial muscles.

The motor nuclei of the other cranial nerves all have bilateral UMN representation, and it is only the part of the motor nucleus of the facial nerve which supplies the muscles of the lower part of the face that has unilateral representation.

A tumour or haemorrhage damaging the upper motor neurones in one cerebral hemisphere produces paralysis on the opposite side of the body. This will principally affect the lower part of the face, arm and leg, producing the upper motor neurone signs mentioned, movements of the muscles which have bilateral representation being unaffected (i.e. movements of the eyes, jaws, upper part of the face, soft palate, neck and tongue).

Dysarthria only results from unilateral upper motor neurone involvement if this causes severe weakness of the facial muscles which control the lips on the affected side. Otherwise disorders of upper motor neurones must be *bilateral* to result in dysarthria, and the causes can be classified as follows:

1 Cerebral vascular lesions.
2 Motor neurone disease.
3 Congenital disorders—e.g. 'spastics'.
4 Neoplasms—e.g. metastases.
5 Miscellaneous—encephalitis, degenerative diseases, severe brain injuries.

For further details of these conditions, see Table 6. Dysarthria due to the disorders of upper motor neurones bilaterally may form part of the clinical syndrome of pseudobulbar palsy.

Table 6 Disorders of upper motor neurones (BILATERALLY) causing pseudobulbar palsy.

	Pathology and aetiology	Signs and symptoms		Treatment
		General	Speech	
1 Cerebral vascular lesions	Arteriosclerosis. Infarction. Haemorrhage. Often associated with hypertension and heart diseases (see Chapter 17)	Often double hemiplegia. Mental condition impaired. Emotional lability. Jaw jerk increased. Spasticity of face. Dysphagia. All may improve	Slurred indistinct articulation. Voice weak (Dysphasia as well if dominant cerebral hemisphere is affected)	Nursing care during acute stages
2 Motor neurone disease	Cause unknown Onset usually in middle age. Progressive deterioration with death usually in 2–4 years (see Chapter 21)	Spastic weakness of muscles, including face, pharynx and limbs. Jaw jerk and limb reflexes exaggerated. Dysphagia. Difficulty coughing. Respiratory distress. LMNs also involved (see Table 4)	Spastic type of dysarthria and dysphonia	Nil specific

Table 6—*continued*

	Pathology and aetiology	Signs and symptoms		Treatment
		General	Speech	
3 Congenital disorders	Environmental and genetic causes. Cerebral palsy (see Chapter 15)	Spastic weakness of limbs, sometimes with 'scissors gait'. Mental retardation and epilepsy often but not invariably associated	Dysarthria, may be staccato or explosive. Specific language defects	Muscular education with relaxation exercises and physiotherapy. Speech therapy and special schooling important
4 Neoplasms	Metastases in both cerebral hemispheres, most commonly from primary malignant tumour in lung (see Chapter 18)	Dependent on localisation of deposits. Raised intracranial pressure (i.e. headache, vomiting and papilloedema)	Dysarthria (may be dysphasia as well)	Radiotherapy in selected cases
5 Miscellaneous	Encephalitis. Degenerative diseases. Severe brain injuries	Mental confusion. Spasticity in limbs. Epilepsy	Dysarthria. Dysphonia	Nursing care, sometimes steroids. Speech therapy and physiotherapy, in suitable cases

PSEUDOBULBAR PALSY

Mechanism of production

Pseudobulbar palsy is not primarily a disease of the bulb but of the corticobulbar fibres (i.e. that part of the upper motor neurone extending from the Betz cells in the motor cortex and terminating in the brain stem at the synapses with the motor nuclei of the cranial nerves).

The term suprabulbar palsy is sometimes used synonymously with pseudobulbar palsy; it is accurate because it implies that the fibres above the bulb are affected and that the lesion is not actually in the bulb. The term pseudobulbar palsy is preferred because it describes the clinical state which resembles bulbar palsy.

The involvement of corticobulbar fibres must be *bilateral* to produce pseudobulbar palsy. This is because not all the corticobulbar fibres cross in the brain stem; some remain uncrossed and continue down on the same side. If the upper motor neurone lesion is unilateral the muscles supplied by the lower cranial nerves are not obviously affected (apart from the lower part of the face) and pseudobulbar palsy will not result.

Clinical features

Dysarthria, dysphonia and dysphagia are the main clinical effects of pseudobulbar palsy. The tone and reflexes of the affected muscles are increased, so there is a brisk jaw jerk, spasticity of the face and exaggeration of the palatal and pharyngeal reflexes. Spasticity in the tongue makes it appear smaller.

In pseudobulbar palsy speech is slow, consonants are indistinct, there are alterations in pitch and phonation, intensity (loudness) is reduced, and speech is nasal. The intervals between sentences and words are longer and the phonemes themselves are prolonged. There is also altered phrasing with grunts at the ends of sentences.

Associated signs

In addition to the bilateral involvement of corticobulbar fibres, the same diseases may affect corticospinal fibres producing upper motor neurone signs in the trunk and limbs with weakness, spasticity (increased tone) and clonus, exaggerated tendon reflexes and extensor plantar responses. There may be impairment of voluntary control of emotional expression, and exaggeration or prolongation of normal responses (i.e. emotional lability with pathological laughter and crying for no apparent reason), causing considerable distress and embarrassment.

Causes of pseudobulbar palsy

The commonest cause of pseudobulbar palsy is *cerebrovascular disease* involving both cerebral hemispheres. Typically there is a history of a stroke (i.e. infarction or haemorrhage) in one cerebral hemisphere (see Chapter 17) followed by recovery and later a second stroke affecting the other cerebral hemisphere. The corticobulbar fibres may have been damaged on the side of the first stroke, but without overt signs because of the bilateral representation. Whether or not there is a residual hemiplegia, the defect of the corticobulbar fibres will not be apparent until the second stroke involves the opposite cerebral hemisphere whereupon pseudobulbar palsy results.

Motor neurone disease can also cause pseudobulbar palsy by progressive involvement of corticobulbar fibres bilaterally. In addition this disease may involve the corticospinal tracts, as well as the motor nuclei of the cranial nerves and the anterior horn cells more or less symmetrically. Thus in some cases, there will be combined features of both bulbar and pseudobulbar palsy, as well as lower and upper motor neurone signs in the limbs (see Chapter 21).

Pseudobulbar palsy may also result from *birth trauma and congenital defects* involving the corticobulbar fibres bilaterally. If corticospinal fibres are also involved, then the pseudobulbar palsy is associated with spasticity of the limbs.

There are other causes of pseudobulbar palsy, such as bilateral *tumours of the brain* (see Chapter 18), e.g. secondary deposits (metastases) in both cerebral hemispheres.

Various combinations of these conditions can cause pseudobulbar palsy; for example a patient may have a tumour in one cerebral hemisphere, and a stroke affecting the other; one hemisphere may be damaged by a head injury, and the other by a vascular lesion or tumour. Pseudobulbar palsy results *only* from *bilateral* lesions of the corticobulbar pathways and the signs are those of upper motor neurone involvement.

DISORDERS OF THE EXTRAPYRAMIDAL SYSTEM

The basal ganglia

These are nuclei of grey matter lying deep in the substance of each cerebral hemisphere. They include the globus pallidus, putamen and caudate nuclei (these three structures constitute the corpus striatum), substantia nigra, subthalamic nucleus (corpus Luysii) and the red nucleus in the upper part of the midbrain. The basal ganglia are the nuclei of the extrapyramidal system. Via connections with other parts of the central nervous system (see Fig. 5), they help to control movement, tone and posture. The mechanism of control is complicated, but diseases of the extrapyramidal system result in involuntary movements and disorders of tone and posture. Involuntary movements include tremor (as seen in Parkinson's disease) chorea, athetosis, ballismus and dystonia.

The disorders of extrapyramidal system which can cause dysarthria are:
1 Parkinson's disease.
2 Chorea—Sydenham's (rheumatic), Huntington's, congenital senile, drug-induced.
3 Hemiballismus.
4 Dystonia.
5 Wilson's disease (hepato-lenticular degeneration).

Parkinson's disease

The tremor of Parkinson's disease is typically coarse and rhythmical, more marked at rest than in action. It usually starts in one hand and, when severe, is classically described as 'pill-rolling'. There may be poverty of movement (hypokinesia) as well as slowness and stiffness of movements of the face which cause a mask-like expression. There are usually defects of fine and associated movements and rigidity of cogwheel type in the limbs. The posture is often stooped and the limbs slightly flexed, the legs shuffling along with small steps (*marché à petits pas*) so that the gait appears hurried or festinant. There is no wasting, the reflexes are unaffected and the plantar responses flexor.

Speech in Parkinson's disease is characteristically monotonous. Rigidity of the muscles of the larynx makes the voice weak and feeble (i.e. dysphonic). Involvement of the muscles used for articulation results in dysarthria. Speech may also be affected in a way comparable to the festinant gait, i.e. words following each other faster and faster, and the same phrase may be repeated over and over again (palilalia). In some patients, excessive salivation or difficulty in swallowing causes dribbling and slobbering which may be exaggerated by tremor of the mouth and tongue (see Chapter 20).

Chorea and athetosis

Chorea usually affects the peripheral parts of the limbs and causes jerky movements whilst the movements of *athetosis* are writhing, and both are purposeless and involuntary.

Athetoid movements are seen in the 'ganglionic' type of cerebral palsy (see page 146) and may be combined with chorea (choreo-athetosis).

Chorea and athetosis cause jerkiness of speech, sometimes with an explosive dysarthria due to sudden involuntary movements affecting respiratory muscles, larynx or mouth, and in severe cases speech is unintelligible.

Hemiballismus

A lesion of the subthalamic nucleus on one side results in hemi-ballismus affecting the limbs on the other side of the body. Ballis-mic movements are involuntary, throwing, purposeless movements, affecting particularly the proximal parts of the limbs, often flinging the limb around violently.

Dystonia

Dystonia is a rare disorder of the corpus striatum, characterised by distortions and bizarre posturing of the limbs and trunk due to spasmodic increases in tone and contractions of muscle groups in a disorderly fashion. It may affect the face and neck or start in one limb and remain localised (torsion dystonia) or become progressively more generalised, and is then called *dystonia musculorum deformans*. Dysarthria, similar to that seen in choreo-athetosis, is sometimes an early feature.

Writer's cramp may be a focal form of dystonia affecting the writing hand, although it has been regarded as a functional

Table 7 Disorders of the extrapyramidal system.

Pathology and aetiology	Signs and symptoms		Treatment
	General	Speech	
1 Parkinsonism			
(a) Idiopathic—*paralysis agitans* (b) Postencephalitic (c) Arteriosclerotic (d) Toxic: carbon monoxide, manganese anoxia, phenothiazine drugs, e.g. chlorpromazine (largactil) (see Chapter 20)	Cogwheel rigidity, tremor, 'pill-rolling' movement of the hands. Shuffling, festinant gait. Expressionless face. Excessive salivation, drooling	Slow with thin, feeble, monotonous voice. Dysphonia. Dysarthria. Rapid repetitions (palilalia)	Drugs (e.g. benzhexol, levodopa, bromocriptine). Neurosurgery (e.g. stereotactic thalamotomy)
2 Chorea			
(a) Sydenham's chorea associated with rheumatic fever	Choreiform movements. Grimacing, fidgeting and dropping things. Other manifestations of rheumatic fever	Speech hesitant and jerky. Dysarthria due to jerky movements of articulatory and respiratory muscles	Rest. Sedation. Salicylates
(b) Huntington's chorea. Age of onset 30–50 years. Familial. Progressive and fatal within 10–20 years	Choreiform movements. Dementia	Dysarthria becoming unintelligible	No specific treatment. Tetrabenazine
(c) Congenital chorea or choreo-athetosis due to agenesis, anoxia at birth, or severe neonatal jaundice—'kernicterus'	Jerky and writhing purposeless movement	Explosive and indistinct. Tongue lacks voluntary control and is overactive. Facial grimacing with continual movements of lips. Irregular spasmodic contractions of diaphragm and other respiratory muscles giving	Motor re-education with special schooling

Pathology and aetiology	Signs and symptoms		Treatment
	General	Speech	
(d) Senile chorea—degenerative disorder of the elderly—not familial	Choreiform movements. No dementia	As above	Tetrabenazine
(e) Drug-induced, e.g. side effect of levodopa (see page 189)	As above	As above	Reduce dose or stop drug
3 **Hemiballismus** Lesion usually vascular, of the subthalamic nucleus (corpus Luysii)	Involuntary throwing, purposeless movements, often violent involving proximal parts of limbs	As above	Tetrabenazine. Neurosurgery (e.g. stereotactic thalamotomy)
4 **Dystonia musculorum deformans** Disorder of corpus striatum, cause unknown, sometimes familial, usually progressive	Distortions and bizarre posturing of limbs and trunk, face and neck may be affected	Same as in choreo-athetosis	None effective
5 **Hepato-lenticular degeneration (Wilson's disease)** Familial, age of onset 10–16 years. Deficiency of copper binding protein, caeruloplasmin, leading to deposition of copper in corpus striatum and liver	Muscular rigidity and involuntary movements. Cirrhosis of liver causing jaundice. Deposition of copper in the cornea of the eye forming Kayser–Fleischer ring	Rigidity of muscles affecting articulation and phonation	Chelating agents (e.g. penicillamine)

(neurotic) disorder and classed as one of the occupational cramps. Muscular spasm, incoordination and discomfort occur only when attempting to write so that writing becomes difficult or impossible. Drug treatment is usually ineffective, but relaxation therapy may help some cases.

Spasmodic torticollis is another condition which may also be a form of focal dystonia causing irregular jerky or sustained torsion of the neck. This again has been thought to be related to psychological factors in some cases, but it may also occur in organic conditions with more generalised involuntary movements.

Further details of the diseases of the extrapyramidal system are given in Table 7, and Parkinson's disease is described in Chapter 20.

DISORDERS OF THE CEREBELLUM

The cerebellum consists of right and left cerebellar hemispheres joined in the midline by the vermis. Each cerebellar hemisphere is connected to the corresponding side of the brain stem by three cerebellar peduncles: (a) superior (brachium conjunctivum), (b) middle (brachium pontis) and (c) inferior (restiform body).

The cerebellum and its connections control the coordination of movements and influence muscle tone. There are important connections with the vestibular mechanisms and cranial nerve nuclei in the brain stem concerned with movements of the muscles of the eyes and neck. The maintenance of balance and coordination of movements are thus dependent upon the integrity of the cerebellum and its connections.

Disturbances of cerebellar function will result in defects of coordination and balance, and affect speech muscles as well as the muscles of the eyes, neck, trunk and limbs.

Cerebellar signs

Defects of one cerebellar hemisphere will cause incoordination in the muscles on the same side of the body (see Fig. 5). Bilateral cerebellar involvement causes generalised incoordination of all limbs, and lesions confined to the vermis affect coordination of the trunk and neck muscles.

Incoordination affecting the upper limbs is seen as 'intention tremor' (i.e. tremor on movement); other signs include difficulty performing rapid repetitive or alternating movements (*dysdiadoko-kinesis*), poor control of the range of movements (*dysmetria*) and clumsiness. Clinical tests used to demonstrate these defects include maintenance of posture of outstretched hands and finger-nose-finger test.

Incoordination affects balance and causes unsteadiness when walking (*ataxia*) so that the patient may veer to one side and tends to sway or stumble. The maintenance of posture and control of movements of the muscles of the neck may be affected so that the head appears to jerk or waver irregularly (*titubation*).

Since coordination of eye movements is dependent upon the connections between the oculo-motor, vestibular and cerebellar pathways, cerebellar lesions are often associated with nystagmus (i.e. a rhythmical involuntary jerking movement of the eyes, usually elicited by asking the patient to look to one side, but sometimes occurring spontaneously when looking straight ahead).

The muscles of articulation may also be affected by cerebellar incoordination, resulting in ataxic dysarthria. Irregularity and incoordination of phonation and respiration add to the difficulty. In mild forms, there is just slurring of speech and the pronunciation of consonants is particularly difficult. Speech becomes slow and thick 'as if there is something in the mouth' and slurring and jerkiness may be combined. Due to poor control of rhythm, there is a tendency to pronounce each syllable as if it is a separate word (*staccato* speech) and to put the emphasis on the wrong syllables, some being pronounced too loudly and others too softly (*scanning* speech). In severe cases speech may become explosive and unintelligible, eventually with complete inability to articulate (*anarthria*).

Diseases of the cerebellum

1 Multiple (disseminated) sclerosis.
2 Hereditary ataxias (e.g. Friedreich's).
3 Degenerations (e.g. idiopathic, carcinomatous).
4 Metabolic and toxic disorders (e.g. hypothyroidism, drugs, alcohol, etc.).
5 Congenital disorders (e.g. dysgenesis).
6 Miscellaneous (e.g. vascular lesions, abscess, neoplasms).

Further details of the disorders affecting the cerebellum are given in Table 8 and multiple sclerosis is described in Chapter 22.

Table 8 Disorders of the cerebellum.

Disease	Pathology and aetiology	Signs and symptoms		Treatment
		General	Speech	
1 **Multiple sclerosis**	Plaques of demyelination scattered throughout the CNS and optic nerves. Irregular course of relapses and remissions. Onset 20–45 years. Females more commonly than males (see Chapter 22)	Optic neuritis. Diplopia. Vertigo. Cerebellar signs: Intention tremor Nystagmus Ataxia. Sensory disturbances. UMN (pyramidal) signs	Slurred. Scanning. Staccato. Dysphasia very rare	Avoidance of fatigue. ACTH for acute relapses. Physiotherapy
2 **Hereditary ataxia**	Friedreich's disease is the commonest affecting cerebellum, cerebellar connections, pyramidal tracts and posterior columns. Associated skeletal deformities (pes cavus, kyphoscoliosis) and cardiac abnormalities. Onset in adolescence, slowly progressive	Cerebellar signs; UMN (pyramidal) signs; posterior column signs; loss of position and vibration sense. Ataxia predominates due to cerebellar incoordination and loss of position sense: absent knee jerks and ankle jerks with bilateral extensor plantar responses	Slow. Slurred. Explosive	Aids for coordination. Physiotherapy, balancing exercises

	General	Speech	
3 Degenerations Idiopathic, cerebellar atrophy. Onset later in life after 40 or 50. Slowly progressive course. No associated skeletal or cardiac disorders.	As above	As above	As above
Carcinomatous degeneration usually associated with carcinoma of the bronchus. Not due to metastases in the cerebellum	Ataxia. Cough, shadow on chest X-ray (sometimes neuropathy as well)	Dysarthria	Nil specific. Removal of primary growth if operable, or radiotherapy
4 Metabolic and toxic disorders Hypothyroidism.	Myxoedema.	Husky voice.	Thyroxine tablets.
Alcoholism	Liver disease. Bilateral cerebellar signs	Dysarthria	Avoidance of alcohol. Vitamin B1
5 Congenital disorders Agenesis or dysgenesis of cerebellum	Oro-facial muscles underdeveloped. Grimacing and drooling. Lack of control of voluntary movement and of posture	Delayed development. Slurred, jerky	Aids for coordination. Physiotherapy, balancing exercises. Speech therapy

Table 8—*continued*

	Pathology and aetiology	Signs and symptoms		Treatment
		General	Speech	
6 Miscellaneous	Vascular lesions, infarction, haemorrhage, often with hypertension. (see Chapter 17)	Mainly ipsilateral cerebellar signs, sudden onset	Dysarthria	Operation for removal of intra-cerebellar haematoma. Nursing care. Speech therapy and physiotherapy during recovery
	Abscess, usually from otitis media (see Chapter 16). Neoplasms (see Chapter 18)	Ipsilateral cerebellar signs, progressive. Raised intracranial pressure	Dysarthria	Antibiotics. Neurosurgery. Speech therapy and physiotherapy following operation on abscess or benign tumour

DISORDERS OF THE CEREBRAL CORTEX

Dysarthria occasionally results from lesions of the motor area which exerts cerebral control over the muscles of the face and those used for speech. This may be accompanied by motor or expressive dysphasia, and results from the same pathological conditions which cause motor dysphasia, for example—trauma, tumour, atrophy, and vascular, granulomatous or other inflammatory lesions (see Chapter 5), the precise form of the speech disorder depending on the site and extent of the lesion.

Unfortunately the terms used (e.g. cortical dysarthria, apraxic dysarthria, verbal apraxia and apraxia of speech) have caused confusion, some implying that the dysarthria is part of the language disorder.

The fact is that dysarthria may coexist with aphasia. The conditions which cause motor aphasia may also interfere with articulation, so that patients can have both aphasia and dysarthria. The cause of this dysarthria is a matter of dispute, but the difficulty with articulation is a purely motor disorder, a disturbance of the programming of the articulatory musculature or an articulatory dyspraxia in contrast to, or in addition to any aphasia which is a disturbance of language. In some cases other movements of the mouth and tongue appear normal when tested individually, but articulatory dyspraxia may also be associated with facial, oral or bucco-lingual apraxia. There are distortions and substitutions of individual phonemes, with signs of groping towards the target word often with difficulty initiating the word, but generally with full awareness of the errors.

DISORDERS DUE TO COMBINED OR DIFFUSE LESIONS

In some cases dysarthria is due to a pathological process involving more than one anatomical level (e.g. in motor neurone disease, both lower and upper motor neurones may be affected causing dysarthria due to a combination of bulbar and pseudobulbar palsy). Dysarthria is also a well-known accompaniment of drowsiness and confusional states when the brain is affected diffusely (e.g. due to inflammatory, metabolic or toxic encephalopathies). Thus drugs and alcohol may produce complex effects on the brain at several levels, disturbing cerebral, brain stem and cerebellar mechanisms serially or simultaneously.

CLINICAL COURSE

The type and severity of the dysarthria vary according to the location and extent of the causative lesion, but the mode of onset and clinical course depend on the nature of the pathological process. For example, dysarthria due to neoplasms and degenerative disorders runs a progressive course whilst vascular disorders typically have a sudden onset with gradual recovery. Fluctuating dysarthria may be due to metabolic disorders (e.g. encephalopathy associated with dialysis or hepatic failure). Transient dysarthria, possibly with dysphasia, is sometimes the aura of migraine attacks; brief recurrent episodes may be due to transient ischaemic attacks or focal epilepsy, and repetitive stereotyped paroxysmal attacks of dysarthria—either alone or with other brain stem disturbances—may occur in multiple sclerosis. Speech becoming increasingly slurred and indistinct during conversation but clear after rest typifies the dysarthria of myasthenia gravis.

Further Reading

DARLEY F.L., ARONSON A.E. & BROWN J.R. (1975) *Motor Speech Disorders*. Saunders, Philadelphia.
NATHAN P.W. (1947) Facial apraxia and apraxic dysarthria. *Brain* 70, 449.

CHAPTER 8
DYSPHONIA

Dysphonia is weakness or hoarseness of the voice due to any lesion interfering with the laryngeal mechanism which governs voice production. There are a variety of non-neurological causes, the commonest of which is a sore throat with inflammation of the larynx (*laryngitis*). Hysteria is also a well-known cause of dysphonia. This is a functional disturbance without structural defect, often a reaction to an emotional upset, particularly in females. These patients usually just whisper and the lack of any true laryngeal disorder is shown by the fact that they can cough normally. Sudden spontaneous recovery takes place when psychological equilibrium is restored.

Patients with a tracheostomy are aphonic as the tube in the trachea prevents the expired air from reaching the larynx. Tumours and local lesions of the larynx also cause dysphonia and the voice tends to become deep and husky in patients with hypothyroidism (*myxoedema*).

The neuromuscular causes of dysphonia

The mechanism of phonation is dependent on the muscles of the vocal cords supplied by the 10th cranial (vagus) nerves (see page 55). The adductors and tensors of the vocal cords contract on phonation and the abductors on inspiration. The vocal cords can be viewed by laryngoscopy and weakness of one or both results in dysphonia.

Dysphonia, like dysarthria, may be caused by the muscle diseases shown in Table 2. In some cases of myasthenia gravis (see page 51) there is excessive fatiguability of the laryngeal muscles which leads to increasing dysphonia, the voice becoming progressively weaker during the course of conversation. After a period of rest without talking or with drug therapy, the voice may recover its strength only to fade again to a whisper after further talking or when the effects of treatment have worn off. This laryngeal fatiguability may be accentuated if accompanied by weakness of the respiratory muscles.

Dysphonia may also be due to lower motor neurone disorders. Those involving the vagus nerve or its branches are shown in Table 3.

The recurrent laryngeal nerve of the vagus is particularly prone to damage in the neck and chest by:

1 Surgery—during thyroidectomy.
2 Carcinoma of the thyroid.
3 Carcinoma of the bronchus and malignant mediastinal growths.
4 Aortic aneurysm.

Occasionally unilateral vocal cord palsy is an isolated phenomenon and full investigation fails to reveal the cause. Some of these idiopathic cases may be due to a virus mononeuropathy of the vagus or recurrent laryngeal nerve.

A unilateral recurrent laryngeal nerve lesion causes paralysis of the vocal cord; the resulting weakness of the voice may be slight and transient due to compensatory movement by the opposite vocal cord. With partial lesions of the recurrent laryngeal nerve. the abductors are always affected before the adductors (Semon's law) and therefore paralysis of adduction cannot occur without paralysis of abduction.

The sequence followed with a progressive lesion is abductor paralysis, midline position of the vocal cord due to overaction of the adductors, 'cadaveric' (intermediate) position and finally compensatory crossing over of the paralysed cord to a paramedian position.

Partial lesions causing bilateral abductor palsies produce laryngeal stridor (a harsh sound from the larynx) during inspiration. Total bilateral paralysis of the vocal cords causes complete aphonia so that the patient can only whisper.

The proximal part of the vagus nerve may be involved in the 'jugular foramen syndrome' in which the 9th, 10th and 11th cranial nerves are affected on one side. This may be caused by lesions at the base of the skull, such as a carcinoma spreading from the nasopharynx.

The lower motor neurone disorders involving the nuclei of the vagus in the medulla are shown in Table 4, and dysphonia is part of the syndrome of bulbar palsy, as has been described in Chapter 7.

Dysphonia is also one of the features of pseudobulbar palsy, resulting from the disorders of upper motor neurones (bilaterally) as shown in Table 6.

Of the extrapyramidal disorders shown in Table 7, dysphonia occurs most commonly in Parkinsonism, when the voice tends to be weak and monotonous. Dysphonia is rarely associated with cerebellar lesions, unless these involve the brain stem as well.

The clinical features and prognosis of neurological (paralytic) dysphonia are dependent on

1 The mode of onset (i.e. acute or chronic).
2 The position of the paralysed vocal cord.
3 Structural changes in the vocal cord (e.g. atrophy).
4 Anatomical variations in larynx (e.g. shape of glottis, position of arytenoids).
5 Compensation of non-paralysed cord.
6 Emotional reactions.

Recovery, dependent on the aetiology, can be divided into five stages:

Aphonia

Following an acute lesion of the recurrent laryngeal nerve (e.g. after thyroidectomy), the patient's voice may be completely lost (aphonia). Noises produced are rough, hoarse, and weak and the patient appears breathless because the period of phonation is reduced, producing rapid breathing (tachypnoea).

Severe dysphonia

Better glottal closure is obtained by compensatory moulding of the cartilages but this is less evident in the elderly (because of calcification).

Flutter voice

With further recovery, the different positions of the two vocal cords produce double tones (diplophony). In some cases, higher tones are lost resulting in a monotonous voice whereas in others, when the glottis is not completely closed, it becomes oval-shaped and results in a high-pitched falsetto.

Mild dysphonia

The volume of the voice increases and the hoarseness is compensated.

Full recovery

Full recovery is dependent on the aetiology and whether residual mobility of the vocal cord has been affected by structural changes.

Further Reading

DRAPER I.T. (1980) *Lecture Notes on Neurology*, 5e. Blackwell Scientific Publications, Oxford.

ROSE F.C. & MURILLO G. (1979) Disorders of Speech. In Scott Brown's *Diseases of Ear, Nose and Throat* p. 539, ed. by J. Ballantyne and J. Groves. Butterworths,

CHAPTER 9
SPEECH AND LANGUAGE DISORDERS
IN CHILDREN

The development of a function depends upon learning processes which necessitate not only the making of new physiological pathways but also the inhibition of irrelevant responses, both at physiological and psychological levels. Learning to read and write involves organising a wide variety of perceptual experiences and motor responses, which may be interfered with by bodily disturbances or brain lesions. In the case of language function, the child has to learn to use these skills for the expression of his own feelings. The learning process is not solely dependent on the acquisition of motor skills and perceptual patterns but also on the structuring of the inner world of the child's mind. This is not a *tabula rasa* but a seething mass of contradictory forces and fantasies, which he must also learn to inhibit when inappropriate. For this reason, it is not surprising that the difficulties of learning methods of communication are often associated with emotional disorders.

A speech defect is a deviation which attracts attention or affects adversely either the speaker or listener. About 10% of children have a speech defect but the incidence becomes less in later age groups. From the age of 6 to 10, 15% are affected but from 10 to 14, this decreases to 5%.

Stammering is one of the common causes of speech difficulty in childhood (see Chapter 10). Less than 10% of the speech defects are due to cerebral palsy and only 1% due to a cleft palate. Ten per cent of the defects are in the sphere of language and only 1% are due to dysphonia.

Speech disorders in children may be due to temporary or permanent interruptions in the normal ontogenetic development of speech (see pages 5 and 6). The majority of children begin to use single words when a year old but the range of normality is wide stretching from 8 months to 2½ years. Words are put together in phrases at about 18 months, again with a wide range from 10 months to 3½ years. In most children, speech is intelligible to the family and friends by the age of two, but one child in three passes through a phase of unintelligible speech during the third and fourth years. Development does not take place at a steady rate; words are used and lost again and there are often silent periods when little progress is made.

The development of speech depends upon hearing and linking of the sounds and symbols of the spoken word. Poor speech development may result from disorders of 'hearing', 'language', or 'articulation' and many children have multiple disabilities.

The development of speech should be regarded as abnormally delayed if the child is not speaking by the age of 3½ years old. If deafness can be excluded (see Chapter 11) the commonest cause of delayed development of speech is mental defect. Information regarding this can be gathered from the child's milestones, e.g.

holding head up	3 months
sitting	6 months
standing	9 months
walking	12 months

Other milestones include self-feeding, being clean and dry, ability to dress, playing alone and character of play.

There may be psychological or emotional causes of delayed speech, and a deprived child may not have the stimulus to speak (e.g. because of being in an institution). With all speech disorders, boys are more commonly affected than girls, and this is particularly so in stammering (see Chapter 10).

The importance of cerebral dominance is controversial in developmental speech disorders but left-handedness and ambidexterity appear commoner both in affected children and their relatives; in one series 5% of normal children were left-handed whereas 50% of the affected children showed signs of cerebral ambilaterality or mixed dominance with a combination of, say, left-handedness and right-eyedness. The failure to establish a completely dominant hemisphere is not necessarily the cause of the delayed speech but may be an associated abnormality of brain function.

CLASSIFICATION

The diagnosis of disorders of speech and language in children can be one of inordinate complexity. Not only does it involve many disciplines but the decision as to whether speech is delayed for pathological reasons can also be difficult. These can be classified into the following disorders:

1   Articulation—dysarthria.
    (a) mechanical (e.g. cleft palate)
    (b) neuromuscular.
2   Voice—dysphonia (see Chapter 8).
3   Language—developmental dysphasia.
4   Reading and writing—developmental dyslexia and dysgraphia.
5   Rhythm—chiefly stammering (see Chapter 10).
6   Secondary to
    (a) deafness—central and peripheral (see Chapter 11)
    (b) mental factors—amentia or subnormality
    (c) psychiatric factors (autism, elective mutism)
    (d) environmental factors (lack of stimulus).

Dysarthria

Disorders of articulation may be due to structural abnormalities of the mouth and jaws, cleft palate, etc, but will not be discussed here.

The neuromusculuar causes of dysarthria in children are best classified according to the anatomical level of the disorders, as in Chapter 7.

Disorders of muscles

Dysarthria may be due to primary muscle diseases affecting the muscles of articulation. These include polymyositis, myasthenia gravis, and the muscular dystrophies. Facioscapulohumeral muscular dystrophy gives a characteristic facies of sunken cheeks with 'snarling grin' or 'tapir mouth'. Dystrophia myotonica is another cause of childhood dysarthria. There is usually a positive family history and the typical story is of drooling, early feeding difficulties, and delayed speech. Examination reveals bilateral facial, neck, and distal limb muscle weakness. Characteristically there is wasting of the sternomastoids and myotonia (that is the inability of muscles to relax quickly after contracting). The tendon reflexes may also be 'hung up' due to delayed relaxation. Even at an early stage cataracts may be discernible on slitlamp examination.

Disorders of lower motor neurones

Bulbar palsy in children. Lower motor neurone lesions include Bell's palsy and bulbar poliomyelitis. Möbius' syndrome is another cause of bilateral lower motor neurone facial weakness. It is due to agenesis of the 7th cranial nerve nuclei and half the cases will be associated with agenesis of the 6th cranial nerve nuclei so that the eyes cannot be abducted.

The dysarthria is of the flaccid type but, since the syndrome may be associated with cleft palate, deafness, and mental subnormality, other types of speech disorder may also be present.

Disorders of upper motor neurones

Congenital suprabulbar paresis. As the name suggests, this is a congenital disorder of the upper motor neurones controlling the 7th, 9th, 10th, 11th, and 12th cranial nerves. It is variable in severity and can be divided into complete and partial syndromes. With the latter the soft palate alone may be affected. More commonly, there is involvement of the facial and lingual movements. In the complete syndrome there is inability to protrude the tongue with involvement of the laryngeal and pharyngeal musculature. Examination reveals a pout reflex and brisk jaw jerk. There is a history of dysphagia and the child is unable to round the lips so that the dysarthria involves particularly the labial sounds and there may be drooling of saliva. One-third of the children have mental subnormality which is more commonly seen in the complete syndrome. Speech improves with age but the drooling may be treated surgically by pharyngoplasty, removal of the submandibular glands or transposition of the salivary ducts to the back of the mouth in children who can swallow fairly well. Medical treatment with atropine-like drugs should be tried first.

Extrapyramidal and cerebellar disorders

Dysarthria in children may also be caused by a lesion in the extrapyramidal or cerebellar pathways, as in the ganglionic and ataxic types of cerebral palsy. Nearly 10 per cent of all speech defects are due to cerebral palsy and different types can be recognized. The ganglionic type talks slowly in a monotonous voice, straining with effort and often substituting difficult consonants. The ataxic type has scanning speech and there is variability in stress and rhythm (*dysprosody*).

Delayed articulation

In early life, as speech and language are being learnt, the initial stages consist of babbling and lalling and articulation takes some years to mature. Although difficulties with articulation occur in the majority of children during speech development, these difficulties persist beyond the age of 5 years in less than 15% of children. Mispronunciations are commoner in social class five. Most cases improve spontaneously.

Prolongation of immature articulation of words beyond the normal age is a form of development dysarthria, that is the retarded or delayed development of normal articulation without any obvious structural cause and usually without any other language deficiency. It is the commonest cause of referral to speech therapists in school clinics.

With this condition children over the age of 5 display immature patterns of speech, perhaps resembling those of a 3-year-old, and may lisp, showing rhotacism (difficulty with the letter r) or sigmatism (difficulty with the letter s). In addition to defective sounds there are omissions and substitutions. Syllables are reversed and the final ones omitted. The last-acquired consonants (that is th, sh, s, b, g, and f) are the most frequently affected. Sounds acquired early in an incorrect manner persist (for example in nursery rhymes). More mistakes are made with spontaneous speech, and such children may also be late in acquiring reading and writing. They may be teased and isolated, and secondary emotional and behavioural disturbances may cause additional problems.

Prolonged observation is sometimes necessary for accurate diagnosis. More severe cases may need special schooling; they should be talked to slowly and clearly. There is no defect in the nervous system apart from the continuing immature speech; lips, tongue, and palate move normally when tested and there is no apraxic difficulty, so there is normally a rapid response to appropriate treatment. This consists of practising the proper pronunciation of words under supervision.

Delayed articulation must be differentiated from the other forms of lalling or idioglossia, in which there is an inability to imitate speech sounds and the response to treatment is less satisfactory.

Disorders of language—developmental dysphasia

There are many different types and several synonyms which lead to confusion. These include developmental dysphasia, congenital auditory imperception, word deafness, audimutitas, idiopathic langauge retardation, developmental speech disorder syndrome (Ingram 1969). Many of the terms suggest an aetiological cause or anatomical substrate which has not yet been proven.

The term developmental dysphasia is paradoxical, in that dysphasia—as strictly defined—is the loss of the ability to express or understand speech after it has been acquired and so differs from disorders of development of speech. The same sort of difference exists between dementia (which is the loss or disintegration of the established mental functions) and amentia (which is the failure of development of mental functions).

The term developmental dysphasia (like developmental dyslexia) is now accepted by common usage and means impairment of language function due to a delay or disorder of development of the cerebral mechanisms. There are many possible causes and the condition is not uncommonly familial. In some there is a history of birth trauma as evidenced by difficult labour, breech delivery, twin pregnancy, forceps or precipitate delivery and prematurity. For the same reasons they may have other manifestations of cerebral palsy. If the left cerebral hemisphere is damaged, the right hemisphere may become dominant, leading to 'pathological' left-handedness. Thus language function may develop normally if taken over by the right cerebral hemisphere, but in some cases speech development is retarded and there may be specific language disorders. Babble is not well developed and this is a significant feature since other milestones may be normal. With diffuse bilateral cortical damage there may be amentia and/or gross disorders of speech and language functions. The speech disturbances may vary from mild distortions of language structure and content to severe degrees of linguistic failure. There may then be overall retardation of language development or a specific language disorder.

In children with developmental dysphasia, the speech defect may be predominantly expressive; most of what is said can be understood especially if spoken slowly, but not in the more severe cases. In others the defect is predominantly receptive and it may be difficult to distinguish this from deafness. In developmental receptive dysphasia the difficulty is in discriminating and appreciating the significance of the sounds heard. The diagnosis cannot be made until the age is reached at which normal children would begin to speak. It should be suspected if the child takes no notice when spoken to and does not repeat words; diagnosis can be difficult because the responses to sound are variable. Audiometry should always be done as the speech defect may be associated with high-tone deafness. This may improve over the years, possibly with conditioning or maturation. Evoked potentials with sound (EEG audiometry) reveal responses in the auditory areas if peripheral deafness is not the primary disturbance.

Routine neurological examination is usually negative (i.e. 'hard' signs such as exaggerated reflexes and extensor plantar responses are rarely found), but special tests may show 'soft' signs (e.g. of motor dysfunction if measured by the Lincoln–Oseretzky test) and these children are therefore sometimes described as having 'minimal brain damage'.

Even in the absence of neurological signs, the aetiology is almost certainly organic, but it is difficult to state 'where' and 'what' the lesion is. The localisation of the lesion is not necessarily the same as the localisation of a function and attempts to understand children's speech disturbances by analogies with adult lesions may be deceptive and unjustifiable. However, the anatomical site of the defect may lie in the inferior parietal lobule (i.e. the supramarginal and angular gyri, Brodmann's areas 39 and 40). This is the 'association area of association areas' upon which projection fibres from the primary motor, sensory, visual and auditory areas impinge. This area is particularly important since speech depends on the ability to form crossmodal associations. The inferior parietal lobule is unique to man (as is speech) and like all recent evolutionary areas in the brain, myelinates late and also forms dendrites late. It is tempting to speculate that this rapidly growing and maturing area is peculiarly sensitive to noxious stimuli and produces the 'disconnection syndrome' of developmental dysphasia.

Although many children with cerebral palsy are mentally defective, this is not invariable since gross neurological (e.g. motor) deficits can occur with little or no impairment of mental or intellectual processes. Furthermore, some children with cerebral palsy have specific defects of motor function (*apraxia*), or sensory function (*agnosia*), of the special senses (e.g. nerve deafness) or of speech and language (e.g. developmental dysphasia, dyslexia, dys-

Table 9　The main headings for a simple clinical assessment of children with speech and language disorders.

1　**Receptive**
　　(a)　Auditory acuity
　　(b)　Reaction to sounds
　　(c)　Pantomime
　　(d)　Speech comprehension with face unseen
　　(e)　Comprehending pantomime
2　**Expressive**
　　(a)　Noises
　　(b)　Words
　　(c)　Pantomime
3　**Reading**

4　**Writing**

5　**Cerebral dominance**

6　**General behaviour**
　　(a)　Interaction with other people
　　(b)　Interaction with animals, objects, tests

arthria). These specific defects can give a false impression of mental retardation, particularly if clinical appraisal is superficial or limited. In order to avoid this pitfall, detailed assessment of speech, language and other cerebral functions is necessary. Tests must of course be geared to the age of the child (see Table 9) and it should be emphasised that a complete and accurate assessment needs a multidisciplinary team including an educational psychologist, neurologist and audiologist, as well as a speech therapist.

If there is a discrepancy between basic intelligence and language function due to defects predominantly in the sphere of speech and language, then attempts should be made to compensate for the specific disorder by special methods of individual training. It is very important that these children as well as those with specific non-language disorders, are recognised and educated appropriately; although requiring patient individual training, many can be helped considerably.

Acquired dysphasia in childhood

This is a different group from developmental dysphasia and may be due to similar pathological processes as in adults, with lesions (e.g.

vascular, infections, tumours or trauma) involving the language area of the dominant hemisphere during early childhood before speech has become fully developed. Other 'hard' neurological signs may or may not be found, depending on the site and the extent of the pathological process. If the lesion affects only the dominant hemisphere, the prognosis for recovery of speech is excellent, and this may depend on the capacity of the non-dominant hemisphere to take over language function. A rare form of acquired dysphasia in children was described by Worster-Drought (1971). In these cases, speech develops normally, i.e. prelinguistic babble is present and two-word phrases and sentences are spoken, but between the ages of 2½ and 6 years, during a period of days or a few weeks, hearing appears to be lost, speech stops, and within a short time these children may become aphasic. Epileptic attacks may occur at, or soon after, the onset. Investigations have failed to reveal the cause although the electroencephalogram (EEG) is usually abnormal, especially over the temporal areas bilaterally; with resolution, these abnormalities—like the fits—usually clear spontaneously over the ensuing few months or years, but the prognosis for language recovery is poor.

A striking difference between the 'developmental' and 'acquired' groups is the sex incidence. The developmental cases, as with specific dyslexia and stammerers, are more commonly boys but the acquired group shows no predilection for either sex. As would be expected, the acquired cases show psychiatric disturbances, e.g. temper-tantrums, mood changes and alteration in personality which may mistakenly suggest a psychogenic aetiology. These are not so common in the developmental group.

Developmental (specific) dyslexia

Loss of the ability to read or write or both in adults is not uncommonly due to a stroke or other cerebral lesion affecting the mechanism that initiates and coordinates the acts of reading and writing (see Chapter 6). Delay in the development of this mechanism in a growing child results in developmental or specific dyslexia which presents special problems, both from the medical and educational points of view. Strictly 'dyslexia' means difficulty in the use of words but has come to be restricted to written words.

There are, of course, many possible reasons for a child having difficulty in learning to read. Those who are generally backward or mentally retarded have difficulty in learning a variety of skills including reading, and visual defects are obviously important. These disorders affect boys and girls equally. However, when delay in the development of the cognitive process in the brain which coordinates the faculties necessary for reading and writing is an isolated functional defect in an otherwise normal person, it is not uncommonly familial (monozygotic twins are invariably both affected) and the condition is 3 times as common in boys as girls.

Although specific developmental dyslexia is regarded frequently as constitutional in origin, it may be multifactorial. The majority have difficulties in the sphere of language, but other sub-types of dyslexia include difficulty copying patterns and diagrams, difficulty with sequencing and various degrees of visuo-spatial-perceptual disorders or word-blindness. Some also have difficulty with writing and spelling, and particularly expressing thoughts adequately with the written word.

The part played by environmental, social and psychological factors has been a matter of much debate, and although the effects of distractability, impulsiveness and poor rapport with teachers may be important influences aggravating or perpetuating the problem, they are thought unlikely to be the primary cause.

The condition is present in about 5% of 10-year-old children, but should be diagnosed between the age of 6 and 9 years. In addition to the frequent family history of dyslexia, there may also be an increased incidence of left-handedness or cerebral ambilaterality.

With regard to the possible genetic influences, just as the tendency to have febrile convulsions in early childhood is often familial, so it is suggested that there may be a familial susceptibility to develop a structural or functional deficit in the *planum temporale*. This is the important association area which has evolved only in man and is larger in the dominant than the non-dominant cerebral hemisphere.

The commonest cause of backwardness in reading is subnormal intelligence with diminution of the overall learning ability. In borderline cases formal assessment of the intelligence quotient by psychological testing is helpful. A difference of at least 2 years between mental and reading ages is probably outside normal limits but because the range of normality is so wide some educationalists have doubted the existence of specific dyslexia.

In some children difficulties arise because they are distractable and restless with poor attention span. This may be due to the syndrome of 'chronic minimal brain damage', which is manifest as backwardness in reading, writing, speaking or clumsy movements, often with a hyperkinetic state or other behaviour disorders. Milestones may be normal but, if delayed, can give an indication of brain damage and there may be corroborative evidence in the history. On psychological testing, visuo-spatial abnormalities are often found so that there is reversal or transposition of letters at a later age than normal. Reading and writing of letters are often much better than of words. There is often an inconsistency in the mistakes, the child at one time being able to read or write a letter or word but not at another time. These children are often able to mirror-write and mirror-read.

Other factors which may be relevant should also be considered (e.g. visual defect, poor teaching with large classes or poor school attendance, and emotional problems).

The various difficulties in reading consist of:
1 Inability to work out the pronunciation of a strange word.
2 Failure to see likeness and differences in forms of words.
3 Failure to see differences in shapes of letters.
4 Making reversals.
5 Failure to keep the place.
6 Failure to read from left to right.
7 Poor concentration.
8 Failure to read with sufficient understanding.

The commonest difficulties found are confusion of letters which have a visual resemblance, such as 'p' and 'q', 'b' and 'd'. More often a child can read the individual letters but makes mistakes with them when reading words. The mistakes made in reading do not differ from those made by a normal child learning to read. The reading speed is reduced and, in addition, the understanding of what has been read is also reduced.

There are often associated writing disabilities, viz. confusion or disfigurement of letters, errors in linking together letters with contamination, mirror-writing, block letters and reversals.

These children may also have (a) disorders of motility, for example dyspraxia, (b) minor sensory disorders, (c) inadequate directional motions, (d) right-to-left confusion with alterations in body image and simultanagnosia (see page 20), and possibly (e) a faulty estimation of time.

Aetiological explanations include the following:

1   A specific lesion near the angular gyrus.
2   Delayed maturation in the parieto-occipital area.
3   Disturbed Gestalt function.
4   Lack of cerebral dominance.

Further Reading

CRITCHLEY M. (1970) *The Dyslexic Child* 2e. Heinemann Medical, London.

FERRY P.C., HALL S.M. & HICKS J.L. (1975) *Dev. Med. Child Neurol.* 17, 749.

FLOW R.M., GOFMAN H.F. & LAWSON L.I. (1965) *Reading Disorders.* F.A. Davis, Philadelphia.

FRANKLIN A.W. (ed.) (1965) *Children with Communication Problems; proceedings of a conference on . . .* Pitman, London.

HALLGRENN B. (1950) Specific dyslexia. *Acta Psych. Neurol.* suppl. 65, 1–287.

INGRAM T.T.S. (1969) Disorders of speech in childhood. *Brit. J. Hosp. Med.* 2, 1608–25.

MYERSON M.D. & FOUSHEE D.R. (1978) *Dev. Med. Child Neurol.* 20, 357.

PECKHAM C.S. (1973) *Brit. J. Disord. Commun.* 8, 2.

RENFREW C. & MURPHY K. (eds) (1964) *The child who does not talk.* Heinemann Medical for Spastics Society (Clinics in Developmental Medicine, no. 13), London.

ROBINSON R.J. (1982) The child who is slow to talk. *Br. Med. J.* 285, 671–2.

ROSE F.C. (1979) *Paediatric Neurology.* Blackwell Scientific Publications, Oxford.

STOTT D.H. (1966) A general test of motor impairment for children. *Dev. Med. Child Neurol.* 8, 523–31.

WORSTER-DROUGHT C. (1971) An unusual form of acquired aphasia in children. *Dev. Med. Child Neurol.* 13, 563–71.

WORSTER-DROUGHT C. (1974) Congenital suprabulbar palsy. *Dev. Med. Child Neurol.* 16, Suppl. 30.

WYNN-WILLIAMS D. (1958) Congenital suprabulbar paresis. *Speech, Pathology and Therapy.* April, p.18.

CHAPTER 10
STAMMERING

There is a vast literature, but little agreement, on the causation of stammering. From one centre alone up to 1955 there were 153 dissertations and 255 publications, and since then the number of reports from all over the world make an analysis of the findings difficult. The main area of dispute is whether stammering is simply an expression of neurosis (the 'psychogenic' theory), or whether it has an organic basis (the 'physiogenic' theory) or whether it is due to a combination of both. There is no doubt that anxiety states occur in many stammerers but whether they are primary or secondary is controversial.

Nomenclature is made difficult because of the use of other terms. Stuttering is the term more commonly used in the United States and some authorities suggest that it is a more severe form of stammering or has a different aetiological background. The two terms are here considered as synonymous.

Definition

Stammering is a deviation of speech which attracts attention or affects adversely the speaker or listener because of an interruption in the normal rhythm of speech by involuntary repetition, prolongation or arrest of sounds. This does not take into account the unreliable judgement of listener or speaker—what is stammering to one person is not necessarily so to another; one speaker may consider that he is stammering when he is not and vice versa. During the development of speech, most children repeat syllables and words (echolalia), and some normal adults stammer under emotional stress, in just the same way as habitual stammerers. In normal children between the ages of two and five years old there is a repetition of words, syllables or phrases about 45 times in every 1000 running words, the upper limit being 100 times per 1000 running words. More than this produces a noticeable stammer.

Incidence

This depends on the age of the series investigated. In children of school age estimates have varied from 0.7% to 4% whereas in adults the incidence is 0.5%. This means that there are about a quarter of a million stammerers in this country and over 15 million stammerers in the world.

Age of onset

Eighty-five per cent of those who stammer begin to do so before the age of 8; there are probably two peaks, namely at about 2–3 years, when the child starts to speak and 6–8 years when the child learns to read soon after starting school and mixing with other children; relatively few start to stammer after the age of 10 years.

Sex incidence

Like speech defects in general, it is commoner in boys; the exact proportion, like its frequency, varies with age. Stammering tends to persist more with boys so that the discrepancy of incidence in the two sexes increases with age. Under the age of 6 years there are twice as many boys as girls affected whilst at all ages there are probably seven times as many males as females affected.

Genetic factors

There is a familial incidence of stammering varying in different series from 36% to 65%. These estimates show a wide discrepancy because of the differences in defining a stammerer and the type of relatives included, e.g. whether only first degree relatives, i.e. parents and siblings are included or more distant relatives as well. The familial incidence does not necessarily imply a genetic factor since environmental factors could also apply to more than one member of the family and, since mimicry is one of the modes of learning in children, imitation is a powerful factor. In families with stammerers, twins are more likely to stammer than the other children. Stammering in some series, but not others, was found to be more common in identical than non-identical twins but, in these cases, the sex incidence does not show the usual male preponderance. Interestingly, the incidence of stammering is greater in families in which twinning occurs than in families without twins.

Stammering occurs more frequently with consonants than vowels in the proportion of about 5 to 1; the vast majority of stammering incidents (96%) are associated with the initial sounds of the word.

Factors that improve stammering are: (a) speaking in unison, (b) modifying the voice by singing, whispering, acting or using a different pitch, (c) repetition of rhymes, stories and choral speaking.

Aggravating factors include emotional states such as anxiety and anger (although this latter sometimes improves it), rapid speech, answering questions and speaking to superiors.

Experimentally, it has been shown that people with normal speech may have their speech disturbed by delayed playback speech (i.e. playing a tape record back through well-fitting headphones with speech delayed 1/10 to 1/5 seconds). With this there is an excessive drawling of vowels with word repetition and stammering. It may be significant that the time period necessary to produce the maximum effect with delayed auditory feedback is approximately the same as the average time period taken for a syllable, viz. 0.18–0.20 seconds. This suggests that the production of speech involves a closed-cycle feedback by which means a speaker continually monitors and checks his own voice production. With delayed feedback, it has been found that when speech sounds are repeated voluntarily, they tend to be continued involuntarily; this can be likened to the facilitation seen in reflex behaviour. Stammering can be almost totally inhibited by interfering with a stammerer's perceptions suggesting that the determining defects are perceptual rather than motor. Auditory perception may be interfered with by deafness or by compelling transference of the speaker's perceptions to a source of sound other than his own speech. Stammering is less common in deaf children.

Shadowing (i.e. copying the speech of another person) is an imitative motor action which often abolishes stammer, presumably because the subject's perception is transferred away from his own voice to the control speaker's voice. Some stammerers have no speech difficulty when singing in a choir or reciting in unison—this is not the same as shadowing because the stimulus is learned. In simultaneous reading, the control could change the text, or even speak gibberish and yet the stammerer continues to read the original text without stammering; this suggests it is not words or the interpretation of semantic concept which exercises control over the stammerer but the sounds themselves, or some elements of the sounds, which may simply act as a distraction.

When a person hears his own voice he hears it by bone and air conduction whereas, in shadowing, he hears it only by air conduction. These pathways differ in their acoustic properties. The stimuli are comparable in loudness but there is a difference in the pitch of sounds transmitted (cf. listening to one's own recorded voice where we hear our own speaking voices at a higher pitch because bone-conducted sounds manifest a low frequency emphasis).

Reflex stammering

Within recent years considerable research has been done on the reflex mechanisms involved in speech. These involve receptors in the larynx, viz. (a) in the mucosa which alter reflexly the tone of vocal cord muscles, (b) in the muscles augmenting tone of opposing muscles, and (c) in the joints which reflexly alter the tone of laryngeal muscles.

These laryngeal reflexes are coordinated with the voluntary action of speech so that the laryngeal muscles are *preset* up to ½ second before the utterance of sound produced by the expiratory air stream. A fault in the presetting mechanism could explain stammering, particularly why it is nearly always initial sounds that are affected and why stammering does not occur with recitation or singing.

Organic stammerers

Electrical stimulation of the brain can produce stammer. Stammer can develop during the course of organic brain disease and differs from habitual stammer in that the sex incidence is equal, and singing or speaking in rhythm or unison will not diminish its severity. 'Organic' stammerers, like habitual stammerers, are worse under stress and may show accompanying facial grimacing and circumlocution. Habitual stammerers have been cured by neuro-surgical operations which have changed cerebral ambilaterality of speech, as evidenced by Wada's test, into a unilateral cerebral dominance (Jones 1966).

Cerebral dominance

Estimates of sinistrality amongst stammerers vary because of differences in testing handedness and footedness, etc. In one series 11% were left-handed and 5% left-sided, as opposed to 6% and 3% respectively in controls.

Earlier reports suggested that the majority of stammerers were cases of shifted sinistrality but this has not been generally confirmed.

Left-handedness is commoner in twins, 10% being sinistrals as opposed to the expected 4%. Over 5% of twins stammer which is more than five times the expected number, and it has been suggested that there was a genetic link between twinning, stammering and sinistrality. Electroencephalography in some cases shows that the alpha rhythm is more symmetrical in stammerers (normally the alpha waves are of lower voltage on the dominant side); this suggests less complete dominance but there is no statistical difference between stammerers and normals.

Imperfect lateralisation for speech indicates lack of cerebral dominance (cerebral ambilaterality) and although this does not imply any psychological abnormality the 'possessor of this type of cerebral organisation is particularly vulnerable to the effects of stress' (Zangwill, 1960). There is little doubt that cerebral dominance for speech is much stronger with right-handed people than sinistrals, i.e. bihemispheric representation of speech is commoner in the latter. In the ambilateral, the proper development of reading and writing, spatial judgement and directional control is relatively easily disturbed (e.g. by brain injury at birth, or by problems in psychological adjustment). A bilingual upbringing, for example, is often noted in stammerers and may be a significant factor in some cases.

It seems likely that stammering has a multifactorial aetiology which includes a constitutional predisposition, incomplete cerebral dominance and environmental factors.

Further Reading

ANDREWS G. & HARRIS M. (1964) *The Syndrome of Stuttering.* Heinemann Medical for Spastics International (Clinics in Developmental Medicine, no. 17), London.
JOHNSON W. (1961) *Stuttering.* University of Minnesota Press, Minneapolis.

JONES R.K. (1966) Observations on stammering after localised cerebral injury. *J. Neurol. Neurosurg. Psychiat.* **29**, 192–5.

PROFERT A.R. & ROSENFIELD D.B. (1978) Prevalence of stuttering. *J. Neurol. Neurosurg. Psychiat.* **41**, 954–6.

QUINN P.T. & ANDREWS G. (1977) Neurological stuttering—a clinical entity? *J. Neurol. Neurosurg. Psychiat.* **40**, 669–701.

RYAN B. (1974) *Programmed Therapy for Stuttering in Children and Adults.* C.C. Thomas, Springfield, Illinois.

TIMMONS B.A. & BOUDREAU J.P. (1972) Auditory feedback as a major factor in stuttering. *J. Speech and Hearing Dis.* **37**, 476–84.

VAN RIPER C. (1971) *The Nature of Stuttering.* Prentice-Hall, Englewood Cliffs, New Jersey.

WYKE B. (1971) The neurology of stammering. *J. Psychosom. Research* **15**, 423–32.

ZANGWILL O.L. (1960) *Cerebral Dominance and Its Relation to Psychological Function.* Oliver and Boyd, Edinburgh.

CHAPTER 11
DEAFNESS

The development of normal speech is largely dependent on the ability to hear, and deafness—if congenital, or acquired in infancy —will delay or prevent normal speech development. In any speech disorder of childhood, it is essential to ascertain whether or not there is any hearing defect.

Hearing is the reception of sound by the ear and should be distinguished from listening which is the act of paying attention to what is heard with the object of interpreting its meaning.

The cochlear system is fully developed by 12 weeks of intrauterine life, although much of the auditory system develops after birth. In the newborn, hearing produces reflex activity, but it does not become discriminatory until about 9 months of age.

There are two main types of deafness:

1 *Conductive*—when the cause is in the ear canal or middle ear.

2 *Perceptive*—when the cause is in the inner ear or involving its central connections; this group can be subdivided into:

  (a) sensory—when the cochlea is affected

  (b) neural—when there is involvement in the neural pathways from the organ of Corti via the 8th nerve, the cochlear nuclei and the ascending tracts to the auditory cortex.

Deafness is of the conductive type in about 40% of cases. Patients with conductive deafness sometimes hear better in noisy surroundings and may speak more softly; those with perceptive deafness tend to confuse speech sounds and may shout owing to difficulty gauging the loudness of their voice. A tuning fork of 512 Hz will be heard better by bone conduction than air conduction in conductive deafness, as opposed to a normal person who will hear it better by air conduction; a patient with perceptive deafness may not hear by bone conduction at all. To be certain of the degree of deafness a quantitative test of hearing such as pure tone audiometry is necessary.

DEAFNESS IN CHILDREN

The prevalence of severe deafness in children, viz. children requiring deaf education, is 1.3/1000. From the point of view of
speech development the age of onset is important. Prior to the
advent of antibiotics, *otitis media* was the commonest cause of conductive deafness in a school child, although it can also result from
eustachian catarrh or just wax in the ear canal (external auditory
meatus). Nerve deafness is an occasional complication of
meningitis or mumps in childhood. The various causes are shown
in the following table:

Table 10   The aetiology of deafness in children

Prenatal

1   Agenesis
    (a) cochlear—familial (with abnormalities of pigmentation = Waardenburg
        syndrome)
    (b) meatal (with failure of facial development = Treacher Collins syndrome).
2   Infections (e.g. rubella (german measles), toxoplasmosis, syphilis).
3   Drugs (e.g. quinine, thalidomide).
4   Endocrine (e.g. cretinism).

Perinatal

1   Birth injury.
2   Anoxia.
3   Prematurity.
4   Kernicterus.

Postnatal

Causing perceptive deafness:
1   Infections, e.g. meningitis, measles, mumps (which may cause unilateral
    deafness).
2   Drugs (e.g. streptomycin, kanomycin, neomycin).
3   Head injury.

Causing conductive deafness:
1   Chronic suppurative otitis media, middle ear effusion ('glue ear').
2   Eustachian tube obstruction (e.g. due to nasal infection or allergy, enlarged
    adenoids).
3   Blockage of external auditory meatus (e.g. by wax, polyp, otitis externa).

Following the onset of deafness after speech has developed (e.g. in a child of 12 years old) speech may continue normally for a time and there may be no noticeable distortions in voice or speech until about a year later. In a younger child whose kinaesthetic patterns are not yet fixed, much earlier breakdown of the auditory monitoring system can occur, and a child of 4 or 5 may show deterioration in speech about 6 weeks after the onset of deafness.

DEAFNESS IN ADULTS

Clinically significant hearing impairment is becoming more prevalent due to an ageing population. Nearly 10% of the adult population in the UK (i.e. 4.2 million) may have a clinically significant hearing disability, defined as an average hearing level in the better ear over the frequencies of 0.5–4.0 kHz which is worse by 35 decibels than the 'normal' standard. Some of these, although not all, will be helped by a hearing aid, depending on the cause and type of deafness, because technological advances allow not only for amplification, modified for each frequency, but also some speech synthesizing to improve intelligibility.

The onset of deafness in adults does not usually interfere with the ability to speak, although there may be some change in the loudness of voice depending on the type of deafness. If a deaf person becomes dysphasic, this will obviously create complicated problems which will need to be analysed and compensated for if possible (Chiarello et al 1982).

There are numerous causes of deafness in adults, some of which are amenable to specific treatment. Those causing *conductive* deafness are the same as in children (see Table 10) with the addition of otosclerosis (see page 102).

The causes of *perceptive* deafness are listed in Table 11, presbyacusis being much the commonest. As far as the other causes are concerned, deafness is either a cardinal feature of a relatively rare condition (e.g. Ménière's disease, acoustic neuroma) or an occasional manifestation of a relatively common condition (e.g. hypothyroidism, Paget's disease).

Table 11 Causes of perceptive deafness in adults.

---

1   Presbyacusis.
2   Ménière's disease.
3   Trauma (e.g. head injury, noise, barometric changes).
4   Acute viral infection (e.g. herpes zoster, mumps).
5   Vascular lesions involving the internal auditory artery.
6   Hypothyroidism.
7   Paget's disease.
8   Neoplasms (e.g. acoustic neuroma, glomus tumour, nasopharyngeal carcinoma, meningeal metastases).
9   Drugs (e.g. aspirin, quinine, streptomycin, frusemide).
10 Hereditary and congenital disorders with late onset of deafness.

Presbyacusis

Some impairment of hearing is expected in the elderly, due to a drop in the higher frequency range. With the changing age profile in the population, people in the present 55–70 age band will survive at a rate such that in 20 years time there will be 700 000 more citizens aged over 75 than we have now, of whom more than half will have a clinically significant hearing problem. Obviously communication will become more difficult as deafness increases, some will learn to lip-read but most should be helped by a hearing aid.

Otosclerosis

This is due to formation of abnormal bone in and around the oval window causing impairment of the mobility of the stapes which results in conductive hearing loss. Otosclerosis is genetically determined and clinically affects 0.5% of the Caucasian population. It occurs twice as frequently in females as in males and is aggravated by pregnancy in one out of four females. Although it is common in Indians, it is rare in Chinese and Negroes. Hardness of hearing is usually first noticed in the second or third decade of life, is frequently bilateral and often accompanied by tinnitus and, occasionally, imbalance. Although a hearing aid may help some, surgical treatment (previously by fenestration of the lateral semi-circular canal or stapes mobilisation, and now stapedectomy) gives very good results.

Ménière's disease

The cause of this condition remains uncertain but is associated with a defect of regulation of the circulation of fluid in the inner ear. This causes slowly progressive deafness with tinnitus and usually incapacitating attacks of vertigo. The latter may be prevented by surgical treatment, but not the deafness. The condition may be unilateral initially, and sometimes continues to affect one side more than the other.

Acoustic neuroma

Progressive unilateral deafness in adults requires careful otological and neurological investigation, in case it is due to an acoustic neuroma. In the past, diagnosis was often delayed until the tumour had compressed and become adherent to the brain stem or cerebellar hemisphere, causing cerebellar signs including dysarthria (see pages 70–4) involvement of the neighbouring cranial nerves—particularly the 7th and 5th—and sooner or later leading to raised intracranial pressure (see pages 168). Although pathologically benign, attempts to remove the tumour required a major neurosurgical procedure carrying a high mortality, and morbidity in those patients surviving the operation.

Nowadays, early diagnosis is possible, firstly by modern audiometric tests (which can differentiate hearing loss due to nerve involvement from that due to diseases of the end organ) and CT scanning. As a result of recent technical advances with the application of microsurgery, total removal of the tumour is often possible by the otologist and neurosurgeon working as a team, using the operating microscope. This method has a much lower mortality and many fewer postoperative problems, with correspondingly good prognosis, highlighting the importance of detecting and investigating cases of unilateral perceptive deafness as early as possible. About 10% of acoustic neuromas occur in cases of multiple neurofibromatosis, and are rarely bilateral.

Deafness resulting from disorders of the peripheral hearing mechanism (i.e. the ear and auditory nerve) must be distinguished from difficulty with comprehension due to receptive dysphasia and mental defects. It is very important that there should be no confusion regarding terms such as word-deafness, cortical deafness and auditory imperception, which describe disabilities of cerebral origin and need different consideration from the usual meaning of deafness, which implies an impairment of the acuity of hearing due to a disorder affecting the peripheral hearing mechanism.

Further Reading

CHIARELLO C., KNIGHT R. & MANDEL M. (1982) Aphasia in a prelingually deaf woman. *Brain* 105, 29–51.
HAGGARD M.P. (1981) What should be done about hearing impairments. *J. Roy. Soc. Med.* 74, 789–92.
MRC INSTITUTE OF HEARING RESEARCH (1981) Population study of hearing disorders in adults: preliminary communication. *J. Roy. Soc. Med.* 74, 189–827.
SMYTH G.D.L. (1978) *Diagnostic ENT.* University Press, Oxford.
WHETNALL E. & FRY D.B. (1964) *The Deaf Child.* Heinemann Medical, London.
WHETNALL E. & FRY D.B. (1964) The young deaf child: identification and management. In Proceedings of a Conference held in Toronto, Canada, 8–9 October. *Acta Oto-Laryngol.* suppl. 206.

CHAPTER 12
MEMORY AND AMNESIA

In addition to the functions of the brain described in Chapter 2, brain activity is reflected by the state of consciousness, which includes awareness, both of oneself and the environment, as well as the capacity to think, learn, speak and control behaviour. An essential common factor for the optimum performance of these functions is the ability to remember. Memory is the capacity to retain experiences and skills and involves reception, registration, retention, recall and reproduction. Each of these processes can be affected independently; for example, reception and registration can be left intact although other aspects of memory are disordered.

Non-specific mechanisms, such as attention and perception, are involved in reception so that memorising is less efficient when the individual is tired or emotionally upset or if attention is distracted by competing stimuli, for example, extraneous noise. The urge to remember depends greatly on the stimulus of interest together with the influence of the emotions such as joy, fear, love and hate. Motivation and concentration also act as important facilitating factors for memorising and successful learning. The word 'memory' is sometimes restricted to the recall of stored material, which is used with ever increasing confidence as the individual matures. Undoubtedly memory mechanisms have an important role in the development of verbal skills, intelligence, mathematical ability, etc., but physiological mechanisms underlying the simplest memory, such as remembering how to walk, are little understood.

An essential part of the physiology of memory is the capacity to repeat previous responses and establish stores of neuronal patterns. Memories have been described as 'facilitated neuronal circuits which never rest'. Repetitive activity probably results in a lower threshold at synapses (see page 53) so that interneuronal communication, dependent on physicochemical changes, becomes more efficient. There are probably separate biochemical mechanisms facilitating shortterm and longterm memory, shortterm memory being accompanied by structural changes in protein whereas longterm memory is associated with protein synthesis and is more stable than shortterm memory. Conditioning of animals produces molecular changes within neurones as evidenced by an increased rate of RNA (ribonucleic acid) neuronal synthesis; conversely, pharmacological inhibition of protein synthesis within the nerve cell can impair the processes of conditioning and learning.

Knowledge and capacity for thought are closely linked with memory for names, words, languages and music, and these are probably stored in the cortex and association areas of the temporal lobe, whereas memory for the motor and sensory skills seems to be a function of the frontal and parietal lobes. All these may be disorganised in lesions causing aphasia (Chapter 5) which may also interfere with the activity of the system whereby memories are preserved. Thought is of little avail without the retention of knowledge, and both recently acquired and long established memories are important for each facet of the speech mechanism, whether it be of sound, sight, the capacity to make a remembered noise in speaking, or movement in writing. It is in this way that the formulation of thoughts and their transfer into words, as well as the ability to learn and judge, have to be integrated with memories derived from events heard and seen.

Many people depend on visual memory, and use of the storage systems is also required when reading. This process includes recognition of the visual patterns of the letters and words and of the associations which add a 'meaning' to the words (although we have little knowledge of what meaning involves in physiological terms). Reading also demands the capacity to remember what is read for long enough to correlate it with later pages. The inability to remember what has been read might be due to a lesion either of the hippocampus or of the storage mechanisms in the posterior parietal lobes.

Retention (the storage of memory) includes organisation and integration and can be improved voluntarily (e.g. by repetition). Recall is the process by which stored memories are brought into consciousness, usually with voluntary effort. Defective recall is usually associated with defective retention and patients may attempt to fill in the gaps in their memory by confabulation, an example of abnormal behaviour accompanying many amnestic states.

Papez (1973) suggested a circuit as the basis for memory integration; this consisted of Ammon's horn, the fornix cerebri, the mamillary bodies, the bundle of Vicq d'Azyr, the anterior thalamic nuclei and the cingulum; between the cingulum and the hippocampal gyrus there are further connections.

The fornix cerebri is the main efferent pathway from the hippocampal gyrus to the mamillary body, but there are fibres in the fornix that arise in other structures and it is estimated that only one-third of the two million fibres in the fornix reaches the mamillary bodies. Although interruption of the Papez circuit has been used to explain defects of memory, this is an oversimplification since bilateral interruption of the circuit need not produce a permanent memory defect; nor does this theory explain memory loss seen in frontal and occipital lesions. Other parts of the brain such as the reticular formation are also concerned in memory function since a state of alertness is important for learning.

Although the *fronto-hypothalamic* system contributes to the emotional drive to remember, it is the *fronto-temporal* neuronal system, particularly in the dominant hemisphere, which facilitates the highly elaborate activity that provides the memory required for speech, thought, initiative and the general control of behaviour. The cortical connections with the thalamus and with the opposite cerebral hemisphere via the corpus callosum are also important so that lesions of these deeply situated structures may also lead to severe disorganisation.

Recently acquired memories are formed from information reaching the sensory receiving areas including the visual and auditory cortex, and there is evidence to suggest that the hippocampus, the fornix of the corpus callosum and the mamillary bodies form a facilitating mechanism for the storage of current events and for the learning of new material. Old established memories on the other hand appear to depend on a different mechanism, maintained by the spontaneous activity of neurones, which is less vulnerable to degenerative and other disease processes. Thus the activity of the hippocampal system which facilitates the storage of current events tends to decline in old age, and this accounts for the forgetfulness of old people who fail to remember day-to-day happenings yet refer accurately to long past events.

Since conscious recall involves using a small sample from a vast mass of experience, most of which have been forgotten, the physiology of forgetting is a relevant consideration. Forgetting is the failure of voluntary recall and may be due to emotional repression; it is probably not a failure to learn but an active process of learning not to remember. Forgotten memories can be shown to be present by the phenomena of dreams, hypnosis, and analysis.

Ribot (1882) first postulated the law of regression in which the ease of retrieval of memories varies inversely with their recency, as happens in normal forgetting—the longer the time since an event occurred the more likely it is to be forgotten. The amount remembered drops steeply in the few seconds and then levels out, but more is forgotten in the first few minutes after an event than in subsequent periods. Ribot also listed successive stages in loss of content; for example, events were first forgotten, then ideas, then feelings and, last of all, actions. In language, proper names were forgotten first, then common nouns, then adjectives, then interjections, and finally gestures. In effect, emotional appreciation in art goes first, then ambition and, last of all, fear and anger. This suggests that there is a gradient from the complex to the simple and from the voluntary to the involuntary.

The clinical assessment of memory is obtained by tests of immediate, shortterm and longterm memory.

Immediate memory

This can be assessed clinically by digit span; normally seven digits can be repeated forward and five digits backwards. The Babcock sentence: 'There is one thing a nation must have to be rich and great, and that is a large, secure supply of wood', can normally be repeated word perfect after three attempts. The span of immediate memory is from 30 seconds to 1 minute and it is characterised by a limited capacity. Disorders of immediate memory produce a failure to retain ongoing events (i.e. anterograde amnesia). Loss of immediate memory can produce disorientation in time and space and, if insight is absent, paranoia.

Shortterm memory

It can be tested by the 'hidden objects' test (in which familiar objects are hidden and 15 minutes later the patient is asked to find them), the capacity for remembering playing cards, and by the 'name, address and flower' test. Whereas immediate memory concerns a span of seconds, recent and shortterm memory has a span of hours or days. Shortterm memories are easily recalled, rapidly forgotten and without permanent record. When shortterm memory is normal, registration cannot be at fault.

Longterm memory

It relates to remote events of a few months or many years ago and has a larger capacity and slower forgetting, being the basis of past learning. When there is a disturbance of longterm memory, it is difficult to decide whether this is due to failure of retention or failure of recall. Since there is no alteration of consciousness, these amnestic syndromes can be distinguished from confusional states.

Mechanisms of shortterm and longterm memory are distinct and differentially susceptible to clinical conditions. This is evident from the striking loss of the ability to store current events while remote memories are conserved, as seen not only in old age as already mentioned, but also in organic brain diseases, particularly with bilateral lesions or after excision of the temporal lobes.

AMNESIA

Amnesia (loss of memory) may be caused by a variety of disorders affecting the brain. Memory impairment is often the first manifestation of a progressive dementia (see Chapter 13). However, many of the following conditions which cause amnesia recover spontaneously or are reversible with appropriate treatment.

Trauma

Amnesia mainly for recent events, and confusion of thought are features of concussion resulting from a head injury (see Chapter 19). In addition to posttraumatic amnesia (PTA), there may also be loss of memory for a period of time leading up to and immediately preceding the impact, and this is called retrograde amnesia (RA). Concussion is due to brain damage which is not macroscopically visible and the resultant amnesia may be due to disturbance of neuronal molecules since, experimentally, concussed guinea pigs show alterations in Nissl substance (which contains RNA). A longer period of PTA occurs with lesions of the dominant left temporal lobe as compared with lesions of the right temporal lobe and other parts of the brain. The ability to remember is regained when hippocampal function recovers or if the hippocampus of the opposite hemisphere takes over.

ECT

Amnesia may occur after electroconvulsive therapy (ECT) which is given for the treatment of depression, and recovery is similar to that seen in posttraumatic cases. Orientation in place occurs before orientation in time and the longest established memories are the first to recover. Names learned early in life return before those acquired later. Shortterm memory and the ability to learn new material usually return within 2–3 weeks, but some deficit may persist for several months. This effect on memory can be prevented or reduced by applying the electric shock unilaterally to the non-dominant cerebral hemisphere.

Encephalopathy

Persistent loss of memory for recent events with retrograde amnesia for months, but retention of memory for long-past events has been reported following *encephalitis* (Rose & Symonds 1960). In this series the patients were unable to remember anything of a current experience even for a space of a few minutes, yet did not show confabulation. One of the four cases in the series has died, and autopsy revealed bilateral atrophy of the temporal lobes.

Local and diffuse brain infections due to various types of encephalitis and tuberculous meningitis (see Chapter 16) can also cause periodic confusion and amnesia which usually clear with recovery from the infection.

Transient amnesia may occur in any severe infection, for example with septicaemia and pneumonia and, on recovery, the patient may have no recollection of the acute state of the illness. Loss of memory and a confusional state may last for minutes or hours and be followed by complete recovery.

Similar transient disturbances may be due to *metabolic disorders*, for example hepatic, renal or respiratory failure, deficiency diseases, drugs and other toxic substances—classic examples being acute alcoholic poisoning and bromide intoxication.

Korsakoff's psychosis and/or *Wernicke's encephalopathy*, often accompanied by peripheral neuropathy, may result from chronic alcoholism which induces deficiency of thiamine and other vitamins of the B group.

Features of the syndrome described by Korsakoff (1887) include loss of memory for recent events, confabulation, confusion with disorientation in time and space, false recognition, lack of insight, and apathy. Vocabulary and previously acquired skills are usually preserved and remote memory, although impaired, is better than recent memory. Characteristic of Korsakoff's psychosis is the impaired ability to acquire new information—anterograde amnesia. Immediate memory is normal but shortterm memory is poor and, on psychometric testing, there is an atypical learning curve with frequent perseveration. Confabulation is frequent in response to questions rather than spontaneous. It is either entirely imaginary or dependent on partial recollections; answers are consistent with the patient's usual activities and occupation but tend to change from one day to the next and consist of 'pseudoreminiscences' (false memories of familiar happenings).

Wernicke's encephalopathy also begins with a global confusional state evidenced by drowsiness, inattention, and disorientation with failure of identification. Nystagmus is nearly always present and ocular palsy, usually incomplete, is present in the majority and delirium tremens in about one-third of cases.

Early treatment with thiamine usually leads to rapid improvement, although the mental disturbances tend to recover only slowly. Amnesia persists for the period of the illness with difficulty in learning and memorising. Retrograde amnesia is rarely complete, the patient retaining islands of information but there is 'telescoping' in which long-past events are thought of as occurring more recently; this incorrect sequencing may partly account for confabulation together with the lack of insight into the amnesia and the associated disorder of perception. In fatal cases the main postmortem findings are focal areas of haemorrhage and neuronal degeneration in the mamillary bodies and mid-brain.

Transient global amnesia

Transient global amnesia is an organic syndrome in which acute disorientation with amnesia of sudden onset lasts for a few hours, although perception and personal identity are preserved. Usually there is complete recovery with a retrograde amnesia that shrinks, although memory of events during the episode does not return. The cause is probably bilateral temporal lobe ischaemia involving the hippocampal regions.

Epilepsy

Transient amnesia is an inevitable component of any attack of loss of consciousness or awareness and so occurs in epilepsy (see Chapter 14). Petit mal consists of transient loss of awareness with amnesia of only seconds after which the child immediately resumes activity or conversation. Retrograde amnesia after a grand mal fit may obliterate the aura and there may also be a period of postictal amnesia with confusion and automatism (inappropriate, fragmented or repetitive behaviour of which the patient later has no memory).

Although postictal amnesia *per se* has no localising significance, automatism is often associated with a focus in the medial part of one temporal lobe. Attacks of temporal lobe epilepsy often involve some memory disturbance, a minority have the classical aura of déjà vu (a sensation of familiarity) or jamais vu (a sensation of strangeness) and the various hallucinations which may also occur can be regarded as forced or distorted memories. These features of temporal lobe attacks mimic or reflect the normal facilitating mechanisms, the epileptic activity stimulating the storage systems concerned with the special senses in the hippocampus (see page 125).

Hysteria

Hysterical amnesia tends to occur in stressful situations, such as domestic disharmony or failure at work. The distinction between this and other forms of amnesia is that the capacity to recall memories still remains, as can be proven using various techniques such as hypnosis or narcoanalysis. Although the memories are beyond voluntary recall they can occur in dreams, or influence behaviour. Hysterical amnesia commonly consists of a 'fugue' lasting for a few hours or even days during which the individual either wanders around aimlessly or makes a specific journey apparently without any sense of identity. Occasionally there is an alternating amnesia in which different episodes are remembered alternately suggesting a 'multiple personality' syndrome. As in normal forgetting, there is resistance to remembering unpleasant events; hysterical amnesia, although subconscious, serves as a defence mechanism and is often associated with anxiety and depression. Recovery, which can either be gradual or sudden, is usually spontaneous, for example when a relative appears, and is frequently associated with a feeling of exhilaration. Hypnosis is only partially successful.

Further Reading

BARBIZET J. (1970) *Human Memory and Its Pathology.* Freeman, San Francisco.

KORSAKOFF (1887) *Vestnik Klin: sudebnoi psickiat-nevropatol.* St. Petersburg (Russian text).

NIELSEN J.M. (1958) *Memory and Amnesia.* San Lucas Press, Los Angeles.

PAPEZ J.W. (1937) Proposed mechanism of emotion. *Arch. Neurol. Psychiat.* **38**, 725–43.

RIBOT T.-A. (1882) *Diseases of Memory.* Appleton–Century–Crofts, New York.

ROSE F.C. (1973) Disorders of memory. *Br. J. Hosp. Med.* **9**, 225–32.

ROSE F.C. & SYMONDS C.P. (1960) Persistent memory defect following encephalitis. *Brain* **83**, 195–212.

ROSE S.P.R. (1968) Biochemical aspects of memory mechanisms. In *Applied Neurochemistry*, eds. A.N. Davison & J. Dobbing. Blackwell Scientific Publications, Oxford.

RUSSELL W.R. (1971) *The Traumatic Amnesias.* University Press, Oxford.

SYMONDS C.P. (1966) Disorders of memory. *Brain* **89**, 625–44.

TALLAND G.A. & WAUGH N.C. (1969) *The Pathology of Memory.* Academic Press, London.

VICTOR M., ADAMS R.D. & COLLINS G.H. (1971) *The Wernicke-Korsakoff Syndrome.* F.A. Davis, Philadelphia.

WHITTY C.W.M. & ZANGWILL O.L. (eds.) (1966) *Amnesia.* Butterworths, London.

CHAPTER 13
DEMENTIA

Dementia means deterioration of intellectual functions, so that there is impairment of memory, intelligence and a wide variety of aptitudes and accomplishments. It is different from amentia, which is the failure or impairment of intellectual development. Mental and intellectual faculties are dependent on the integrated and selective functions of the millions of cells in the cerebral cortex. The greatest degree of *learning* ability is in youth although, with experience and training, memory patterns and skills are established and judgement improves. During middle life, the cells of the cerebral cortex begin to dwindle, probably by more than a 100 000 each day. This is part of the natural process of ageing (physiological senescence) so that most old people do not have the same intellectual capacity as when they were young, the earliest sign being loss of memory for recent events with a tendency to become forgetful of names. Physiological senescence and senile dementia are not synonymous as dementia implies a pathological process.

If intellectual deterioration occurs before the age of 65, the term *presenile dementia* is used, but this serves only to indicate the relatively early age of onset as the pathological causes may be the same as in the elderly. The disruption of mental functions is often generalised (global dementia) and includes deterioration of intelligence, memory, behaviour and personality. Deficits can also be selective, so that formal intelligence may be preserved yet serious lapses of judgement occur.

The development of slovenliness may occasionally be an important early feature of dementia, but there is usually failure of memory and of the power of reasoning, lack of retention or recall, and loss of learning ability. Often the presenting problem is a slowing down or loss of efficiency at work, an increasing inability to perform professional duties with failure to complete the usual tasks. This may be accompanied or followed by disorientation or confabulation and perseveration.

Depression is sometimes a symptom of dementia but occasionally severe depression resembles dementia and must be differentiated because it may respond to antidepressant treatment, whereas the other manifestations of dementia do not. Likewise focal cerebral lesions which cause frontal lobe disinhibition, dysphasia and parietal lobe syndromes with apraxia must be distinguished, although they may also coexist with dementia. If the dementia is severe, confusion and disorientation may be accompanied by delusions and hallucinations. There may be epileptic attacks and a variety of neurological signs, often with incontinence. In some, there is irritability, restlessness and aggressive or antisocial behaviour, whereas others have a state of apathy, withdrawal or euphoria. The presenting features often seem to be dependent more on the premorbid personality than the pathological process.

Patients who complain that they have to write notes as they are unable to remember things, usually do not have any serious disease. Their subjective forgetfulness may not be confirmed by tests and may be due to an anxiety state or neurosis, not infrequently associated with headache and lack of concentration. The patient with organic dementia, in contrast, often conceals or is unaware of his disability and, lacking insight and judgement, may have to be persuaded to consult a doctor.

The description by relatives and friends of changes in behaviour and personality together with the findings on clinical examination will usually indicate that the deterioration in mental and intellectual abilities comes into the category of dementia.

Examination of the mental state

It is necessary to observe general behaviour, for example, relationship to other people and the response to situations and the surroundings.

Tests for memory and intellectual deterioration should include the assessment of orientation in space and time, simple arithmetical tests, such as 100 minus 7, sentence repetition, and tests of general knowledge. Obviously these tests need to be geared to the intellectual background of the individual patient.

The patient's method of speaking as well as the content should be observed and sometimes taped, particularly spontaneous talk, which may be hesitant, slow, or discursive with sudden changes of topic.

The patient's mood and the presence of delusions or hallucinations should be noted, as well as whether the patient is orientated as to his own name, identity, place, time and date.

Memory for both recent and more remote experiences can also be assessed as can the grasp of general information, insight and judgement. The patient should be asked to write something in his own time, for example a brief account of a day in his life.

The Babcock sentence, 'There is one thing a nation must have to be rich and great, and that is a large, secure supply of wood', is a useful test. It is repeated alternately by the examiner and patient until the patient says it perfectly. Normally this is achieved within two or three attempts; failure after several attempts is indicative of dementia. Gross perseveration of an error is typical of an organic intellectual loss, and fragmentary repetition is suggestive of a language defect. Gross variability in response is often characteristic of psychoneurosis (Zangwill 1943). The explanation of simple proverbs is another useful test.

Types of demented speech

In any patient with dementia—whatever the cause—speech may be affected. Usually there is poverty of speech; in some, vocabulary becomes limited early, in others it may be preserved until quite late in the illness. There is difficulty in retaining series but, unlike aphasic patients, paraphasia, neologisms and portmanteaux words do not occur. Names for objects are often not completely accurate although they may have a close association. Interjections are rarely used although speech can be exclamatory. Speech is simplified consisting of statements, descriptions or requests, often of no importance, and in severe cases there is a failure to communicate.

It has been found that the ratio between the numbers of verbs and adjectives used varies, as in neurotics, and there is also variation in the length of sentences and punctuation. The frequency of the pronoun 'I' is also of interest: used in 5% of words over a telephone by a normal person it is used in 0·01% in technical speech. Both in dementia and aphasia sentences are started but not finished (*aposiopesis*) and there is filling in with unnecessary additions (*paralogisms*). Perseveration is extremely common; words are used normally but then reiterated and this also occurs in writing (*echographia*). Dysphasia may co-exist with dementia if the language area is involved. In Pick's and Alzheimer's disease, speech is slow and there may be interpolation of the 's' and 't' sounds, and the voice also tends to become higher-pitched.

A demented patient has difficulty in understanding quick or noisy speech. Gesture, gesticulation, mime and mimicry may all be impaired, possibly in part due to slowness of movements (*akinesia*). The term *alogia* has been used for the impoverishment of speech in dementia; this differs from the purely communicative defects of dysphasia, which is due to a local lesion of the specific area of the brain concerned with speech. Although speech therapy will not help if there is a significant degree of dementia, it is important to be aware of the different types of altered speech observed and the pathological processes of the brain which interfere with the mental faculties.

Causes of dementia

Dementia is not a diagnosis but a manifestation (cf. dysphasia and hemiplegia) of various diseases; the classification shown in Table 12 is suggested.

The term dementia has been used in the past to imply an irreversible state as the pathological causes were nearly always progressive or untreatable. This is no longer invariably the case, since several of the causes of dementia can now be treated effectively (e.g. benign intracranial tumours, vitamin B12 deficiency and neurosyphilis). Early diagnosis of these treatable conditions is important as the degree of recovery depends largely on how early treatment is started.

Investigations of dementia

All patients with dementia require investigation to establish the cause as soon as possible, particularly to identify those that are treatable. Various blood tests will reveal some of the causes, and examination of the cerebrospinal fluid and electroencephalography are useful in some cases. The development of CT scanning has been particularly helpful for the diagnosis of intracranial disorders. As it is a non-invasive procedure, it has largely superseded the traditional neuroradiological techniques such as arteriography and air encephalography. It shows intracranial tumours (indicating not

Table 12   Causes of dementia.

Metabolic disorders

Deficiency of vitamin B1 (Korsakoffs' psychosis, Wernicke's encephalopathy, see Chapter 3), vitamin B2 (pellegra) and vitamin B12
Hypothyroidism
Hypoglycaemia
Hepatic and renal failure
Drugs (e.g. barbiturates, alcohol, bromides, arsenic, lead, mercury)
Cerebral anoxia (e.g. following cardiac arrest)
Lipidoses

Degenerative diseases

Alzheimer's, Pick's
Huntington's chorea
Creutzfeldt-Jakob disease

Cerebrovascular disease

Multiple infarcts, arteriosclerotic dementia
Binswanger's encephalopathy

Infections (see Chapter 16)

Neurosyphilis

Hydrocephalus (see Chapter 15)

Obstructive, Communicating

Tumours (see Chapter 18)

e.g. of frontal lobes and corpus callosum

Trauma (see Chapter 19)

Brain injuries
'Punch drunk' syndrome
Chronic subdural haematoma

---

only their position but often their pathological type as well) and cerebral atrophy. In the latter, the cortical sulci are widened and the ventricles dilated due to the degenerative changes and shrinkage of the cerebral substance. Dilatation of the ventricles without widening of the cortical sulci signifies hydrocephalus, which if 'communicating' in type (see Chapter 15) may be relieved by a shunt procedure. The CT scanner will also show chronic subdural haematoma and other vascular lesions.

Further Reading

BEHAN P.O. (1982) Creutzfeldt–Jacob Disease. *Br. Med. J.* **284**, 1658–9.

LEADING ARTICLE (1980) Alzheimer's Disease. *Br. Med. J.* **281**, 1374–5.

LEADING ARTICLE (1981) Binswanger's encephalopathy. *Lancet* i, 923.

LISHMAN W.A. (1978) *Organic Psychiatry*. Blackwell Scientific Publications, Oxford.

PEARCE J. & MILLER E. (1973) *Clinical Aspects of Dementia*. Bailliere Tindall, London.

ROSE F.C. (ed.) (1981) *Metabolic Disorders of the Nervous System*. Pitman Medical, Tunbridge Wells.

CHAPTER 14
EPILEPSY

The word 'epilepsy' is derived from the Greek and means seizure. The disorder is one of the oldest recorded, being referred to in the Hammurabi laws of Babylon 4000 years ago, as well as in the Bible and in the writings of Hippocrates. Its ancient name was 'the Sacred Disease', and in England it was called 'the Falling Sickness'. In the last 100 years, attacks with loss of consciousness and convulsions have been distinguished from minor lapses of awareness or 'absence' by the French terms grand mal and petit mal respectively, but now petit mal has a more specific meaning (see page 123) and there is a tendency to refer to any epileptic attack as a fit or seizure.

Definition

Epilepsy is the liability to recurrent epileptic attacks (seizures), the outward effects of transient disturbances of brain function taking many different forms, often but not invariably with loss of consciousness. The many functions of the brain include speech, memory, thought, attention and behaviour, the performance and coordination of movements, and the perception, recognition and interpretation of sensations, and so a great variety of epileptic attacks can result from disturbances of one or more of these functions. There are many medical conditions which affect the brain and lead to epileptic attacks, so that epilepsy, like headache, is a symptom of the underlying cause. It is not a single disease and so the modern tendency is to talk about 'the epilepsies' rather than 'epilepsy'. Those with recurrent epileptic attacks due to a known cause are said to have *symptomatic epilepsy*, but in many cases no underlying structural or metabolic abnormality is ever found, and the epilepsy is then called *idiopathic*.

TYPES OF EPILEPTIC ATTACK

The normal activity of brain cells is associated with electrical discharges but, in those with epilepsy, abnormal or excessive discharges occur during attacks, and in some cases between attacks. These electrical discharges (normal and abnormal) can be recorded using a machine called an electroencephalograph (EEG). When an abnormal electrical discharge arises in the brain, the nature of the epileptic attack will depend firstly on the area of the brain affected and the function that it normally controls, and then on the extent to which the discharge spreads to involve other areas of the brain. Bring primarily cerebral in origin, the attacks consist of disturbances of consciousness, movement, feeling or behaviour. They are transient and paroxysmal, ceasing spontaneously but liable to recur in a stereotyped pattern (i.e. the same sequence of events recurs in each attack in a given individual). Diffuse and bilateral disturbances and involvement of the deeply situated parts of the brain cause loss of consciousness; if a small superficial area of one cerebral hemisphere is involved, the attack affects one or more specific functions. It is because the brain has such a complex structure and controls such a variety of functions, that many different types of epileptic attacks can occur. Nevertheless for practical purposes, epileptic attacks can be classified into two main categories: generalised and partial (focal) (see Table 13).

Table 13. Types of epileptic attacks.

1 Generalised
   (a) grand mal (tonic-clonic)
   (b) petit mal
   (c) myoclonic

2 Partial (focal)
   (a) simple partial
   (b) Jacksonian
   (c) complex partial (e.g. temporal lobe)
   (d) partial becoming generalised

GENERALISED EPILEPTIC ATTACKS

Generalised epileptic attacks may
(a) occur as a primary phenomenon (i.e. the seizures result from an intermittent disturbance of the cerebral hemispheres which is diffuse and bilateral from its onset)—these are *primary generalised seizures.* There is no evidence of any underlying disorder between attacks. This is idiopathic epilepsy. The attacks may be of grand mal (tonic-clonic) type, petit mal or myoclonic and occasionally status epilepticus may occur
(b) result from diffuse or multifocal disorders of the cerebral hemispheres (e.g. encephalitis)—these are *secondary generalised seizures*
(c) result from a focal cerebral disturbance, when a partial seizure discharge spreads centrally to involve both cerebral hemispheres—this is described as a *partial seizure with secondary generalisation.*

Grand-mal (tonic-clonic) seizures

The typical grand mal epileptic attack (major seizure) starts with sudden loss of consciousness and the patient may fall. There may be a brief warning or aura immediately beforehand if the fit starts as a partial seizure and then becomes generalised. At the onset of the attack there is often a cry or grunting noise due to the involuntary expulsion of air through the closed glottis indicating the start of the *tonic phase* (i.e. sustained stiffening of the body with the arms and legs held rigidly in flexion or extension). The patient may make gurgling, groaning or choking sounds, and froth or foam at the mouth if saliva oozes out. This may be blood-stained if the tongue or inside of the mouth has been bitten as the jaw is clenched. Breathing becomes heavy (stertorous) and may cease temporarily causing congestion and blueness (cyanosis) of the face due to asphyxia. The tonic phase lasts for about half a minute and is followed by the *clonic phase,* i.e. alternating contractions of the extensor and flexor muscles of the limbs causing violent rhythmical repetitive jerking movements (i.e. convulsions), which may last for a few minutes. During unconsciousness, the bladder and occasionally the bowel may empty (incontinence) and injuries may result from falling as consciousness is lost. Consciousness usually returns within a few minutes, often with a stage of confusion and irritability, and sometimes with automatic behaviour (*automatism*) which is not remembered. During the postictal phase the patient may complain of headache, muscular pains and nausea. Others may vomit and remain drowsy for a while, but recover completely after sleeping for a variable period of time.

This is the typical grand mal or *tonic-clonic* seizure, but not all epileptic attacks are so dramatic and there are many variations. Sudden loss of consciousness is the cardinal feature but either the tonic (stiffening) or clonic (jerking) phases may predominate. Sudden loss of muscle tone may cause the individual to fall to the ground and sustain injury, so called *drop attacks* (atonic seizures). Some have a few brief jerks of the limbs, head or body (*myoclonic epilepsy*) which may be followed by loss of awareness.

Petit mal

Petit mal is another type of primary generalised epilepsy; it almost invariably begins in childhood and is idiopathic. The attacks consist of brief interruptions of awareness—'absences'—lasting for just a few seconds at a time. The child's mind goes blank and expression appears vacant usually with the eyes open and staring, but sometimes with the eyelids flickering. He may miss part of a sentence, so losing the thread of conversation, without any other outward sign that anything is amiss. This may lead to his being accused of inattentiveness or daydreaming (e.g. at school). Occasionally he may drop things or even fall momentarily but recovery is rapid. These attacks can recur several times a day or even several times in the course of a few minutes. When very frequent, for example 100 per day, the name *pyknolepsy* is given, but this is a rare disorder.

Petit mal attacks are associated with a characteristic pattern of generalised electrical discharges on the EEG. These consist of high voltage bilaterally synchronous discharges of spike-wave complexes recurring regularly at 3 cycles per second (Fig. 7). This EEG picture differentiates true petit mal from other forms of absence and minor epilepsy where loss of consciousness is also incomplete or momentary but due to focal cerebral disturbances.

Partial (focal) epileptic attacks

These seizures result from disturbances in localised areas of the cerebral hemispheres, the type of attack depending upon which area is affected. A focal lesion (i.e. disease or injury affecting a localised area of brain) may, for example, cause recurrent attacks of jerking of one foot, lasting for a few seconds without loss of consciousness. In the current international classification of epileptic attacks, this would be called a 'simple partial seizure'. If the causative lesion is progressive (e.g. a brain tumour), this is likely to lead eventually to a permanent deficit, and in such a case the foot and then the leg may gradually become paralysed. Focal electrical discharges may remain localised and then cease spontaneously, but sometimes they spread to contiguous areas of the cerebral cortex. This spread or 'march' of the abnormal electrical discharges is reflected clinically; for example attacks may start with jerking in the right foot, then involve the whole leg, then the hand and face on the same side, possibly followed by transient dysphasia and tingling on the right side of the body. This indicates that the electrical discharge started in the leg area of the motor cortex of the left cerebral hemisphere, spread rapidly downwards to the face and speech area and then posteriorly to the sensory cortex. This type of focal epileptic attack, lasting for only a few seconds, with the sequential spread or march of the electrical discharge is called 'Jacksonian epilepsy'. The focal discharge may also spread to the central areas of the brain and involve both cerebral hemispheres resulting in a generalised seizure. This is then called a partial seizure with secondary generalisation.

'*Complex partial seizures*' are a form of focal epilepsy where attacks originate from an abnormality in one frontal or temporal lobe, causing absence or loss of awareness, with disturbances of behaviour, memory, speech, hearing and/or of the senses of smell, taste, vision and balance. Epileptic attacks involving the temporal lobes have been called *temporal lobe epilepsy*. If the focus lies in the speech area of the dominant cerebral hemisphere, the attacks may consist of transient dysphasia. Others may have brief distortions of memory, e.g. the patient may just for a few seconds relive experiences that occurred sometime previously, or feel that he is seeing or doing something which seems familiar but which he may not have seen or done before (*déjà-vu*, *déja-fait* phenomena); or everything may seem strange and unfamiliar when it is in fact well known to him (*jamais-vu*). Odd sensations known as 'dreamy states' may occur, as well as the feeling of not existing (depersonalisation and derealisation). The patient may be aware of a smell, often with a burning or musty nature or indescribable. With this or separately, he may experience a peculiar, indescribable or perhaps familiar taste. These hallucinations of smell (olfactory) and taste (gustatory) usually last just a few seconds and are due to a lesion of the uncus (the medial part of the temporal lobe) and are called *uncinate attacks*.

Various other hallucinations also occur:

Auditory: the impression of hearing a sound, such as bells ringing, phrases from a musical theme or voice which may or may not be familiar.

Vertiginous: the sensation of rotatory movements, either the head spinning or the room going round and round, similar to that experienced when getting off a roundabout.

Visual: formed hallucinations of vision may consist of remembered scenes, familiar objects, places, people or faces and all sorts of fictional images. There may be distortions of visual perception, e.g. seeing objects as smaller (micropsia) or larger (macropsia).

If visual hallucinations consist of crude (unformed) but stereotyped phenomena, for example, various shapes or abstract patterns which are not recognisable or remembered as particular objects, or flashing lights appearing in homonymous parts of the visual fields, then the epileptogenic focus is likely to be situated more posteriorly in the temporo-occipital region, closer to the visual cortex.

Attacks of temporal lobe epilepsy may thus consist of recurrent disturbances of speech or memory, or one of the above hallucinations, lasting for a few seconds at a time. Others may lose awareness for a short time with abnormal or automatic behaviour (*automatism*). This may include repetitive movements such as chewing, champing the lips or swallowing, picking at clothes or even undressing, and walking around aimlessly with no recollection of any of these events (i.e. *psychomotor attacks*) which may be mistaken for psychiatric disturbances.

If the focal discharge in the temporal lobe spreads to become bilateral and generalised, then a grand mal seizure results, and the preceding transient disturbance is then the aura of the major seizure. The aura is of course part of the attack, but is very important because it localises the focus of origin or epileptogenic focus (e.g. an aura of a peculiar smell or taste indicates a temporal lobe origin, whilst an aura of jerking of the right leg would indicate a focal lesion irritating the motor region of the left cerebral hemisphere). Some auras resulting from focal lesions in the temporal lobes are less distinct consisting of abdominal sensations, a sickly or sinking feeling in the stomach (visceral or epigastric aura) which may move up to the head and be followed by loss of consciousness. In others there is just an indescribable sensation in the head (cephalic aura). If there is no aura because the electrical discharge so rapidly becomes generalised with loss of consciousness, or if the patient fails to remember the aura subsequently, evidence of a focal origin may still be obtained from investigations, for example an electrical focus may be found on the EEG (see Fig. 7), or a cerebral tumour or an angioma demonstrated by X-rays.

Causes

No one fully understands the mechanism causing fits, but they are accompanied by sudden abnormal discharges of electrical activity in the brain. Integrated action of the various parts of the brain depends upon a balance of excitatory and inhibitory impulses transmitted to and from different groups of cells throughout the brain and controlled by neurochemical substances. Anyone with a normal brain may have a fit or convulsion at any age under certain circumstances, as from a powerful electric shock, administration or withdrawal of certain drugs, or if the brain is injured. In some individuals, fits result from an increased sensitivity to certain stimuli, such as a high fever in young children (febrile convulsions), rapidly flickering lights (photic sensitivity), and may even be provoked by profound degrees of emotional stress and lack of sleep, as well as by a variety of toxic and metabolic conditions, including excessive alcohol and fluid intake. The susceptibility or threshold to fits varies in different individuals, and may vary in the same individual at different times. Genetic or constitutional factors influence the liability to have fits, some brains being more susceptible than others. There is a wide range of factors which provoke fits (Table 14).

Attacks resembling epilepsy, sometimes with convulsions, may result from conditions which do not arise primarily within the

Table 14   Factors provoking fits.

Hyperventilation
Photic and other reflex stimuli
Stress, sleep deprivation
Metabolic factors
    (e.g. overhydration, premenstrual state, fever, hypoglycaemia, hypocalcaemia,
    uraemia, alcohol, drugs, or their withdrawal)
Structural brain lesions—focal and diffuse

---

brain. These include cardiac causes of syncope, certain conditions causing a fall in blood sugar (*hypoglycaemia*) or in blood calcium (*hypocalcaemia*) and renal failure with uraemia. The diagnosis in these cases is that of the underlying systemic (extracranial) disorder of which the 'epileptic' attacks are symptomatic and secondary. Often the seizures will cease when the primary disease has been dealt with effectively.

In children, epilepsy may be due to congenital or developmental abnormalities of the brain (e.g. resulting from maternal infections damaging the fetal brain *in utero*, or birth injury). Epilepsy may also result from injury to the brain at any time (posttraumatic epilepsy) or may be a symptom of any other structural cerebral lesion. Epilepsy starting in an adult (i.e. after the age of 20) is referred to as 'epilepsy of late onset' and is more likely to be symptomatic. Although brain tumours are a well-known cause of epilepsy, only about 20% of late onset cases do in fact have a cerebral tumour and some of the remainder will turn out to have idiopathic epilepsy in spite of the late age of onset. Epileptic attacks with focal features in adults nearly always have a structural cause and require special investigation. Brain disorders causing epilepsy (see Table 15) may be single focal lesions (e.g. *angioma, abscess*), multifocal, scattered lesions (e.g. *metastases*) or diffuse disease (e.g. degenerative, inflammatory). All have the tendency to increase the excitability of nerve cells in such a way that they may give rise to abnormal electrical discharges, but not everyone with a damaged or diseased brain will have epileptic attacks. Only about 50% do, which suggests that there are inhibitory factors preventing clinical attacks, as does the fact that a small proportion of people have EEGs with abnormal discharges yet do not have fits. Of all the

Table 15   Aetiology of epilepsy.

Idiopathic
Constitutional

Symptomatic
Tumours
Infections (e.g. encephalitis, abscess, neurosyphilis)
Cerebral infarction
Trauma
Toxic and degenerative diseases
Congenital malformations, angioma

---

known causes of epilepsy, one which has become more common but could be prevented is head injury from road traffic accidents. The wearing of seat belts can not only save the lives of many of those involved in accidents but may prevent them from sustaining head injuries and the subsequent brain damage which may lead to epilepsy. Motor cyclists are also particularly vulnerable to accidents and sometimes sustain head injuries which can result in epileptic attacks.

Idiopathic epilepsy

In the majority of people who have recurrent generalised epileptic attacks, there is no evidence of a structural abnormality of the brain nor of any disease elsewhere, the attacks occurring spontaneously or with only slight provocation. The attacks are the only clinical manifestation of the brain disorder which is intermittent with normality between attacks.

There is an increased susceptibility to have seizures or an inherently reduced threshold, possibly a defect in the inhibitory mechanisms, so that there is a failure (albeit intermittently) to control the excitatory impulses. This may be genetically determined (i.e. inherited) and so account for the small familial incidence of epilepsy, although direct inheritance of the epileptic tendency is not common. Presumably there is an abnormality at a cellular or metabolic level that cannot be defined by the present techniques of investigation.

The EEG in idiopathic epilepsy typically shows paroxysms of abnormal generalised excessive electrical discharges, bilaterally synchronous, originating either diffusely from the cerebral cortex or from structures deep in the cerebral hemispheres or from the reticular substance of the brain stem.

Attacks due to primary generalised epilepsy usually start in late childhood, are relatively easy to control and tend to diminish in frequency or cease spontaneously in adolescence or early adult life. It has to be distinguished from *secondary generalised epilepsy* which is due to focal or multifocal areas of diseased or damaged brain and more difficult to treat, often being associated with mental and physical handicaps. The brain damage may occur early on in life, but the cause is not always evident.

Status epilepticus

A series of fits occasionally follow one another rapidly so that the patient has hardly recovered from one when the process is repeated (serial epilepsy). 'Status epilepticus' of grand mal type occurs when the fits recur repeatedly without any intervening recovery of consciousness. This is a dangerous condition which may prove fatal, intravenous administration of drugs is usually necessary, and so all such cases should be admitted to hospital for appropriate treatment as soon as possible. Focal fits which continue unabated for long periods are referred to as *epilepsia partialis continuans*.

Speech disturbances in epilepsy

With petit mal, the attacks may interrupt the child's normal flow of speech, he may miss something that is said to him and lose the thread of conversation during the transient period of loss of awareness.

In partial epilepsy when the focus lies in the dominant hemisphere attacks may have a dysphasic aura; with an epileptogenic lesion in any part of the speech area, the attack itself may consist only of transient dysphasia or there may be a dysphasic aura preceding a grand mal seizure. The dysphasia may consist of any of the disturbances of speech and language described in Chapter 5, and such transient dysphasia—either alone or as the aura of a grand mal attack—is of great localising value indicating that a lesion lies in the speech area of the dominant cerebral hemisphere.

Dysphasia or hemiplegia discovered for the first time *after* an epileptic attack may be the result of the epileptogenic lesion, but such signs occurring postictally do not always have the same localising significance as the aura, as they may be due to an inhibitory effect of the fit (Todd's paralysis). Recovery from this usually takes place within a few days.

ELECTROENCEPHALOGRAPHY

Electrical activity in the human body is a reflection of the biochemical and metabolic processes of individual cells. The electrical impulses from the brain were originally recorded by Berger, a German psychiatrist who published his first paper in 1929. The impulses generated are the sum total of electrical activity of the 10 000 million cells of the cerebral cortex and can be recorded by multiple electrodes applied to the scalp and amplified by a machine called the electroencephalograph (EEG). The predominant pattern of the normal alert adult EEG consists of alpha or Berger rhythm of 8–13 cycles per second (Fig. 7a) which is recorded chiefly over the occipital areas. The alpha rhythm is more marked when the eyes are closed and becomes less prominent with the eyes open (blocking of the alpha rhythm). In people with epilepsy, the abnormal and excessive electrical discharges can also be recorded by the EEG not only during attacks, but in some cases (although not all) between attacks as well. The recordings may thus provide useful information about (a) the type of epilepsy, as the pattern of the abnormal electrical discharges varies in different types, and (b) the localisa-tion of the origin of the epileptic attacks, which may be shown if the electrical abnormalities recorded are focal (i.e. confined to two or three adjacent electrodes—see Fig. 7b).

During the recording of the EEG, subjects are usually asked to overbreathe (hyperventilate) and to look at a rapidly flickering light (photic stimulation), each for a short time, as in sensitive subjects these may provoke electrical abnormalities which have not been evident otherwise.

In primary generalised epilepsy, the interictal EEG often shows paroxysms of bilaterally synchronous sharp complexes of high voltage (see Fig. 7c). Fig. 7d shows spike-wave complexes of petit

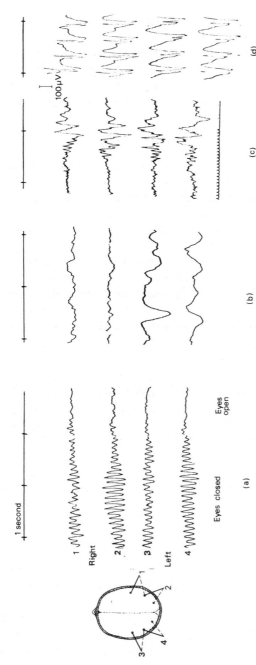

Fig. 7 Electroencephalograms. (a) Normal record in an alert adult; alpha rhythm blocking when eyes opened. (b) Left posterior parietal tumour; focal abnormality with slow waves. (c) Idiopathic epilepsy; bilateral sharp wave discharges provoked by flicker. (d) Petit mal; 3 c/s spike and wave complexes.

mal. In some cases these abnormalities may be provoked or exaggerated by hyperventilation, photic stimulation (flicker) and occasionally by other special techniques when recording the EEG. In others, although undoubtedly having epilepsy, the EEG recorded between seizures is not infrequently normal but this does not exclude either idiopathic or symptomatic epilepsy; even brain tumours do not always show abnormalities on the EEG. The EEG may show focal abnormalities (Fig. 7b) which reflect a local lesion of the brain such as a tumour or abscess, but as a rule no conclusion regarding the pathological nature of brain lesions can be made from the EEG alone. About 10% of normal people (i.e. who have never had a fit) have an abnormal EEG, so that whether or not a person has epilepsy is not as a rule dependent on the electrical findings, but on whether the person has attacks recognisable clinically as epileptic.

Recently developed electronic techniques using telemetry and ambulatory monitoring enable the EEG to be recorded for pro-longed periods; this increases the chance of visualising the electrical abnormalities during a seizure, and the clinical features of the seizure can also be analysed by video filming at the same time as the telemetric recording of the EEG.

DIAGNOSIS

A single seizure or convulsion does not constitute epilepsy if there is no clinical, EEG or other evidence of an underlying cause, nor if provoked by exceptional circumstances. If there is such evidence following a single seizure, or if a second attack occurs without some exceptional provocation, or if unexplained attacks recur, then there is a liability to recurrent attacks, which is indicative of epilepsy.

Isolated or recurrent attacks of loss of consciousness may, however, be due to causes other than epilepsy (e.g. syncope, i.e. fainting). This has a different mechanism from epilepsy, being due to transient impairment of the blood supply to the brain. It is usually easy to distinguish from epilepsy, although not always. As a rule when someone has recurrent attacks of loss of consciousness, a thorough medical examination and investigations will be necessary.

TREATMENT

The treatment of epilepsy is a specialised subject and can only be touched upon here. Many aspects of the care of the patient have to be considered besides treatment with drugs. There are now several anti-epileptic drugs which are often effective particularly if carefully selected according to the type of epilepsy (see Table 16).

In the last few years, laboratory techniques have made it possible to measure the concentration of anti-epileptic drugs in the blood. When fits are not controlled, if the blood sample shows that the concentration of the drug is below the optimum range, the doctor may suspect that the drug is not being taken as prescribed, or if it is, that the dose is inadequate and needs to be increased. On the other hand a very high concentration of the drug in the blood may confirm that the dosage is too high and may be causing toxic side effects, which require reduction of the dosage. This has proved to be an important advance, enabling the doctor to adjust the dose more efficiently and reduce the danger of side effects.

The aim nowadays is to prevent attacks with one drug (monotherapy) taken regularly. If the drug chosen is not effective in spite of increasing the dose and achieving an optimum concentration of

Table 16   Anti-epileptic drugs in common use.

	Petit mal	Grand mal	Partial (focal) seizures
Ethosuximide (Zarontin)	+		
Sodium valproate (Epilim)	+	+	
Carbamazepine (Tegretol)		+	+
Phenytoin (Epanutin)		+	+
Phenobarbitone (Luminal)		+	+
Primidone (Mysoline)		+	+

Table 17   Drugs used for status epilepticus (given intravenously).

Diazepam (Valium)
Clonazepam (Rivotril)
Phenytoin (Epanutin)
Chlormethiazole (Heminevrin)
Paraldehyde

the drug in the blood, then a second drug may be tried. This should be given preferably instead of the first drug rather than in addition to it, although some cases are still treated with two or more drugs. Tables 16 and 17 show the drugs in common use for the various types of epileptic attacks.

Treatment of a grand mal attack

The patient having a fit should not be moved unless in danger from traffic, fire or other hazard. Something soft should be put under the head, and the head turned to one side. It is rarely possible to prevent the tongue from being bitten; this certainly should not be attempted with fingers, and nothing should be forced between the teeth (the tongue will heal but broken teeth will not).

The unconscious person should not be left lying on his back or unattended. As soon as possible after the convulsion, he should be turned onto his side, so that any saliva or vomited material drains out of the mouth and not into the lungs which could have serious consequences. The airway has to be kept clear, dentures removed if possible and the collar loosened. Recovery usually ensues without any complication and it is only necessary to call for an ambulance or a doctor if a serious injury has been sustained or if a series of convulsions develops (*status epilepticus*). Medical advice should be sought following the first fit and for optimum control of established epilepsy.

Surgical treatment of epilepsy

If the causative lesion is, for example, a benign tumour, surgical removal may be possible and would offer a high chance of cure, although epileptic attacks may still recur due to residual brain damage. Computerised tomography (the CT scan) is a major technical advance for the X-ray demonstration of structural intracranial lesions.

If repeated EEGs in patients disabled by epileptic attacks intractable to medical treatment show a consistently focal electrical abnormality in an area of the brain which can be excised (e.g. the anterior part of one frontal or temporal lobe), neurosurgical treatment is occasionally possible even when special X-ray investigations have failed to reveal a lesion.

Removal of the anterior 5–6 cm of one temporal lobe, sparing the superior temporal gyrus, is called *temporal lobectomy*. Such operations are suitable for a small proportion of those with temporal lobe epilepsy whose attacks prove resistant to medical treatment. Pathological examination of the removed tissue sometimes shows *mesial temporal sclerosis* or atrophy (shrinkage) with gliosis which is considered to be due to hypoxia resulting from birth trauma or prolonged convulsions in infancy.

Other neurosurgical procedures have recently been devised for the treatment of intractable epilepsy but cannot yet be regarded as established. These include stereotactic procedures and implantation of a stimulating device into the cerebellum.

SOCIAL ASPECTS

Throughout the ages, epilepsy has been the object of many superstitious beliefs. For centuries people with epilepsy were thought to be unclean, mad or possessed by the devil—misconceptions which even today linger on, so that those labelled as 'epileptics' still suffer from stigma. In the 19th century people with severe epilepsy were often kept in lunatic asylums, although in no sense mad. Later, colonies were established so that people with epilepsy were cared for while taking part in the work of a small self-contained community, although the trend was still to segregate them in institutions. Only in recent years have medical advances made it possible to control attacks, and enlightened attitudes enable the majority to live at home. Even with severe cases the aim now is to look after them within the family circle whenever possible, leaving just a minority that are so intractable and have such unsatisfactory social circumstances that permanent care in a special centre is the only solution.

Unfortunately there is still a tendency to refer to children and adults who have epileptic attacks as 'epileptics'. Someone with quite infrequent attacks (e.g. once a year) or even free from recurrence perhaps for several years and having no other disability, may still be labelled 'epileptic'. Whereas people with diabetes can without harm be called 'diabetics', two people with epilepsy are so rarely alike, there are so many different types and causes of epilepsy, with all degrees of severity and frequency, that it is unhelpful to call them 'epileptics'; worse still, it conjures up the mediaeval misconceptions that many people still have about epilepsy and perpetuates the stigma. *The attacks may be epileptic but not the person.*

Epilepsy can start at any age, it most commonly does so in childhood and often before the age of 20 years. It can affect people of every kind regardless of their previous state of health, income group, educational level or social background. Famous people said to have had epilepsy include St. Paul, Socrates, Julius Caesar, Alexander the Great, Napoleon, Dante, Byron, Handel, Tchaikowsky, Dostoevski and Alfred Nobel.

About five per 1000 of the population have epilepsy in one form or another. This means that in England and Wales there are about 300 000 with epilepsy, about a third of whom are children. Most people with epilepsy can marry and have children, but no one with epilepsy should withhold the information from his or her prospective partner. The situation should be fully discussed together and preferably with their families and medical adviser. The question of the risk of any children of such a marriage inheriting epilepsy should also be discussed with a specialist in the genetic aspects. The actual risk will depend on several factors, but particularly on the cause of the epilepsy. If epilepsy due to certain rare diseases of the brain can be excluded and if only one of the partners has epilepsy, then the risk of their children having epilepsy is relatively small, albeit greater than if neither parent had epilepsy.

The appearance of someone having a major fit is undoubtedly unpleasant and frightening. With treatment, however, attacks can be controlled in the majority; about a quarter will derive some benefit from treatment but will also have some continuing difficulties and restrictions to face. The remaining quarter or possibly less—as not all patients cooperate or comply fully with the advice given—are not really helped by treatment. Some (albeit the minority) have associated physical, intellectual or psychiatric handicaps which, like the epilepsy, are manifestations of the underlying disorder of the brain. Some certainly react to the social difficulties, which they may have had to suffer from childhood onwards, by developing a variety of behaviour and personality complexes. The majority of people with epilepsy have no mental or physical disability, apart from their propensity to have fits, and many difficulties experienced arise from public attitudes and misconceptions. While most handicaps arouse a certain amount of sympathy, people with epilepsy often encounter prejudice, hostility and rejection, which may cause as much distress as the epilepsy itself. People can come to terms with their attacks but the prejudice of others makes this condition one of the most difficult to suffer, and may interfere with education, employment and social activities. Unfortunately employers are still prejudiced against taking on someone with epilepsy. Obviously some types of jobs are unsuitable, especially where attacks put others at risk (e.g. aeroplane pilot, driving, working at heights, operators of certain types of machinery, train driver, etc) but many jobs and most of the professions can be undertaken, except by the most severe cases. Even though attacks may be infrequent, obvious risks to the person who has epilepsy should be avoided in case an attack occurs, and the safety of others must be protected, but excessive restrictions should be avoided; they may be unnecessary and unfair. Where reasonable attitudes have prevailed, there is no evidence that those with epilepsy pose a serious risk of accidents at work. Each case must be considered individually—the nature, severity, timing, frequency, and degree of control of attacks on the one hand, and the suitability of the job on the other.

With regard to the regulations under the Road Traffic Act concerning applicants for driving licences who have had epileptic attacks, recent amendments allow granting ordinary licences to those with a history of epilepsy under the following conditions:

1   If free from attack for 2 years.
2   If attacks have occurred only while asleep over a period of at least 3 years.
3   If the driving of a vehicle is not likely to be a source of danger to the public.

Many people with epilepsy are now able to lead useful and active lives in spite of their condition. This does not mean that there are no difficulties, but often these can be overcome. It is vital to understand that epilepsy is a physical disorder which is not something to be ashamed of, and sufferers should not be shunned or scorned.

Further Reading

HOPKINS A. (1981) *Epilepsy: the Facts.* University Press, Oxford.

LAIDLAW J. & RICHENS A. (1982) *A Textbook of Epilepsy*, 2e. Churchill Livingstone, Edinburgh.

MCGOVERN S. (1982) *The Epilepsy Handbook.* Sheldon Press, London.

MCMULLIN G: P. (1981) *Children Who Have Fits.* Duckworth, London.

OFFICE OF HEALTH ECONOMICS (1971) *Epilepsy in Society.* Office of Health Economics, London.

ROSE F.C. (1982) *Research Progress in Epilepsy.* Pitman Medical, Tunbridge Wells.

SCOTT D. (1978) *About Epilepsy*, 3e. Duckworth, London.

TEMKIN O. (1971) *The Falling 'Sickness*, 2e. Johns Hopkins Press, Baltimore.

PART 2

CHAPTER 15
CONGENITAL MALFORMATIONS AND CEREBRAL PALSY

Congenital malformations are defined as abnormalities of structure present at birth. Infant mortality has decreased since the beginning of the century from 130 to nearly 20 per thousand live births; this progress is a reflection of improvements in antenatal and obstetric care together with advances in medical treatment of neonatal disorders. The number of children with congenital diseases has not changed so that they now provide a considerably higher proportion of neonatal mortality: whereas in 1900, 1/30 of the neonatal mortality was due to congenital abnormalities, now the proportion is approximately 1/4.

The incidence of congenital malformations depends on what is taken to be a malformation, whether stillbirths are included and the age at which the incidence is assessed. It is approximately 1.5% at birth, increasing to 5% at the age of 1 year. In a recent study of the outcome of pregnancies lasting 28 weeks or more in 22 977 women in Scotland and England, there was an incidence of malformations in 2%. The definition of malformation was 'a malformation evident at birth or within 6 weeks in either a live or stillborn infant which could be diagnosed unequivocally excluding skin malformations'. A further 1.9% had abnormalities including skin malformations and a selection of equivocally diagnosed problems.

The CNS is the commonest system affected by congenital malformation, 50% of all congenital lesions being neurological. Of 15 cases with congenital abnormalities, three will have spina bifida, two anencephaly, two hydrocephalus, two heart disease, two cleft palate, and two Down's syndrome (mongolism). The next commonest are club feet and dislocation of the hip. At least seven of the 15 have CNS involvement, or more if any of the cases of Down's Syndrome are mentally defective or retarded as they often are. Other congenital conditions associated with mental defects include microcephaly and agenesis of the corpus callosum. 70% of all cases of severe mental retardation are due to disorders occurring in the prenatal period. About 1/3 are due to chromosomal abnormalities of which Down's syndrome is the commonest. Single-gene disorders account for 7% of all cases; these include neurocutaneous syndromes such as tuberous sclerosis and neurometabolic conditions such as phenylketonuria.

AETIOLOGY OF CONGENITAL MALFORMATIONS

The causes may be environmental or genetic.

1 Environmental causes acting on the fetus via the mother include:
   (a) dietary lack, either of protein, vitamin A, riboflavin, folic acid or thiamine
   (b) hormonal deficiency, e.g. of pituitary, thyroid or pancreas
   (c) drugs, e.g. thalidomide, cortisone, antibiotics, nitrogen mustard, anticonvulsants
   (d) physical agents, e.g. radiation, hypoxia, hyperthermia
   (e) infections, e.g. rubella (german measles), toxoplasmosis, syphilis.

2 Genetic causes include chromosome mutation which may affect many systems (e.g. Down's Syndrome) and gene mutation which usually affects only one system.

The type of congenital defect depends on the stage of development of the fetus when the damage occurs. Severe malformation of the CNS such as anencephaly, hydrocephalus and spina bifida cystica occur in about 1/150 births.

Anencephaly. It is due to a defect of the closure of the embryological neural tube, the brain is virtually absent, and this is usually incompatible with life. It occurs in females more than males in the proportion of 5:1 and is often associated with an absence of the ganglion cells of the retina. There is a geographical variation in incidence (e.g. it is three times commoner in Ireland than in London).

Hydrocephalus. This is due to excessive accumulation of cerebrospinal fluid (CSF) within the cranial cavity and occurs in about 1/1000 births. The CSF is formed by the choroid plexuses, which consist of a mass of tangled capillaries and lie in the lateral, third and fourth ventricles. By a process of selective perfusion and filtration, the CSF is produced from the plasma in the choroid plexuses, passes through the foramina in the roof of the fourth ventricle into the subarachnoid space, and is absorbed via the arachnoid villi into the dural venous sinuses.

Hydrocephalus is described as *obstructive* if the circulation of the CSF is blocked in the third ventricle, aqueduct or fourth ventricle; an example is aqueduct stenosis (which can be inherited in a sex-linked recessive manner). The lateral ventricles dilate and the cerebral cortex becomes thin.

Communicating hydrocephalus occurs when the CSF is not adequately absorbed from the subarachnoid space, which may be due to adhesions following meningitis.

The head circumference is normally 33.1 cm at birth, 36.8 cm at one month, 39.4 cm at two months and 46.8 cm at a year. A hydrocephalic head is abnormally large and globular in shape with protuberance of the forehead, bulging fontanelles and prominent scalp veins. There is a cracked-pot note on percussion of the skull. These are the effects of excessive CSF under high pressure, occurring before the sutures of the baby's skull have fused. About 50% of cases arrest spontaneously and 25% reach adult life. The average IQ of hydrocephalics is 70, but 10% have an IQ above average. One-third have no physical disability, but the others tend to have squints or various degrees of spasticity. Frequently there are other associated abnormalities present as well (e.g. an *Arnold–Chiari malformation*).

In the *Arnold–Chiari malformation* the medulla is elongated and extends into the upper part of the cervical canal with prolongation of the cerebellar tonsils which are also herniated through the foramen magnum. The cisterna magna is obliterated, the circulation of CSF is obstructed and so results in hydrocephalus.

Hydrocephalus may also be associated with *spina bifida*, in which there is a developmental defect of the spines of one or more vertebrae, which is sometimes combined with failure of closure of the neural tube, resulting in a *meningo-myelocoele*. In these complicated cases the prognosis is poor.

Microcephaly (abnormal smallness of the head and brain). This occurs in approximately 1/1000 births; it is always associated with mental deficiency, and a third of the cases have epilepsy. Similar complications are associated with *agenesis of the corpus callosum*.

The development of language functions are likely to be delayed, or will remain retarded and immature when there are severe mental and intellectual defects.

CEREBRAL PALSY

Cerebral palsy is not a specific disease but is the term used to cover a variety of non-progressive disorders of the brain resulting from maldevelopment, injury or disease and presenting in early infancy. Children with cerebral palsy may be classified on the basis of one of the following:
1 The type of movement disorder (e.g. spasticity, dyskinesia, ataxia).
2 The topographical picture (e.g. diplegia, tetraplegia, hemiplegia).
3 Aetiology (e.g. kernicterus, anoxia, birth injury, infection).

The abnormalities of brain function are reflected most obviously by defects of movement, often but not always with failure of development of intellect, speech and language, and disturbances of behaviour and emotional control. In many of the children affected, the limbs are stiff and there are pyramidal signs; this is the group often referred to as 'spastics'. In 10% of cases involuntary movements of an athetoid type—and not spasticity—constitute the principal disability, while in about 5% of cases, the limbs are actually hypotonic and the child may be clumsy and ataxic rather than spastic. All grades of severity are encountered; at one extreme, cerebral palsy merges into minimal cerebral dysfunction, at the other into profound mental retardation with severe educational subnormality and physical handicap.

There is difficulty in assessing the distribution and size of the problem (i.e. the incidence and prevalence rates). This may be due to variations (a) in definition and recognition of the syndromes, (b) in completeness of ascertainment of cases. This also depends on the age of children included in the ascertainment (e.g. the prevalence is less in surveys of children between the ages of 0 and 4 than in those between 5 and 15 years old, as the problems increase and may only come to light when the child goes to school). A decrease in the incidence (i.e. of new cases) may also be masked by improved survival rates which will lead to an increase in prevalence. However, the survival rate of low-birthweight babies (i.e. of 4 lb = 1814 g or less) has not only improved greatly over the last 20 years, but is also associated with a decrease in handicap from cerebral palsy. The incidence of cerebral palsy is approximately 7 per 1000 births; of these one dies in infancy, two are mentally defective, one is severely handicapped, two can be rehabilitated, and one has only mild disability. It is the latter two groups that are the most important from the point of view of speech therapy. Between one and two of every 1000 schoolchildren have some form of cerebral palsy.

The majority of cases of cerebral palsy are congenital, i.e. due to prenatal or perinatal causes, but some result from postnatal conditions occurring in infancy.

Aetiology of cerebral palsy

Prenatal

1 Effect of maternal disorders on fetus *in utero*:
   (a) anaemia or toxaemia of pregnancy
   (b) infections transmitted from mother, e.g. rubella (german measles), toxoplasmosis, syphilis
   (c) rhesus incompatibility.
2 Other embryological defects:
   (a) agenesis
   (b) porencephaly.

Perinatal

1 Prematurity (low birth weight).
2 Birth trauma.
3 Anoxia due to prolonged labour or difficult delivery.

Postnatal

1 Infection (e.g. encephalitis).
2 Cerebral venous thrombosis.

The proportion of children with cerebral palsy due to birth trauma has probably declined and more attention has been focussed on the possibility of agenesis or hypoagenesis (i.e. a failure of development of part of the brain which occurs for reasons usually unknown). Anoxia during or shortly after delivery accounts for some cases.

Rubella (german measles) if contracted by the mother during the first three months of pregnancy, is particularly liable to cause congenital malformations.

During embryonic life, the primitive organs go through phases of rapid development at different times, during which they are vulnerable to infection. The stage of development of the fetus at the time of infection will determine which embryological structures are likely to sustain maximum damage and, presumably, the severity of virulence of the infection is also significant. The common congenital malformations which result from rubella are deafness, congenital heart disease, abnormalities of the eyes, and occasionally more serious defects such as anencephaly.

Rhesus incompatibility may cause serious defects of the fetus. This is dependent upon the mother being rhesus negative and forming antibodies which on mixing with the fetal circulation, interfere with the maturation of fetal red blood cells resulting in varying degrees of *erythroblastosis fetalis*. The effects range from anaemia to severe degrees of jaundice which may produce *kernicterus* where bile pigment is deposited in the basal ganglia, and sometimes more diffusely throughout the brain, causing the ganglionic athetoid type of cerebral palsy, often with mental deficiency and deafness. The level of maternal antibodies increases with succeeding pregnancies so that the degree of erythroblastosis increases with each baby born; two or more such pregnancies may result in a miscarriage or still-birth. Modern methods of treatment will now prevent fetal damage.

Clinical types of cerebral palsy

Although cerebral palsy usually reveals itself by a delay in development with failure to pass the intellectual and physical milestones at the appropriate age, most cases fall into a number of distinctive clinical syndromes.

Spastic

This is the commonest variety of cerebral palsy with upper motor neurone signs affecting the limbs, e.g. spastic diplegia (Little's disease), monoplegia, hemiplegia or double hemiplegia; this may be associated with mental defect varying from slight mental retardation to amentia and many of these cases develop epilepsy.

The mildest cases show a delay of a few months in learning to walk with some clumsiness and unsteadiness of gait, symmetrical exaggeration of the lower limb tendon reflexes and extensor plantar responses. Often the child is unable to walk until the 5th or 6th year and then does so with a characteristic 'scissors gait' due to spasticity of the adductor muscles; contractures tend to develop in the tendo-Achilles and posterior thigh muscles. In the most severe case, walking never becomes possible and all four limbs are spastic, indicating bilateral or diffuse involvement of corticospinal pathways.

If the left cerebral hemisphere is maldeveloped or damaged, the right hemisphere may become dominant, leading to 'pathological' left-handedness. Language function may develop normally (e.g. if taken over by the right cerebral hemisphere) but in some cases speech development is retarded and there may be specific language disorders (see Chapter 9). With diffuse bilateral cortical damage causing amentia, speech and language functions may fail to develop.

Dysarthria is either due to a localised cortical defect causing articulatory apraxia or more commonly to pseudobulbar palsy resulting from bilateral involvement of corticobulbar fibres.

Athetoid

This is sometimes called the ganglionic or extrapyramidal type due to involvement of the basal ganglia or other parts of the extrapyramidal system. It produces disorders of tone and posture with involuntary movements (e.g. athetosis or choreo-athetosis). These movements are not apparent until the 2nd year of life or even later, although the limbs are hypotonic and movement is incoordinate. Some cases have associated spasticity.

Speech in these cases is grossly distorted with an explosive dysarthria; there may also be dysphonia or interference with intonation and facial grimacing.

Ataxic

This type is due to involvement of the cerebellar hemispheres and produces various degrees of incoordination and hypotonia, often with nystagmus. The speech disorder is due to an ataxic dysarthria.

Various combinations of the above clinical types occur, and there may be associated defects, e.g. deafness (which occurs in about 25% of cases, most commonly in the athetoid group), squint (strabismus) or other visual defects.

The age at which the diagnosis is made depends upon the severity of the condition, but it is usually within the first 12 to 18 months of life; in others, delay and difficulty in walking are not apparent until later in the 2nd year. The diagnosis of mental defect in early life, depending as it does on failure to achieve new milestones of intellectual development at the normal age (e.g. smiling, following a light, groping for objects, forming syllables and words, etc.) requires experience because of normal variations.

Although a large proportion of patients with cerebral palsy are mentally defective, this is not invariable since gross neurological (e.g. motor) deficits can occur with little or no impairment of mental or intellectual processes. Furthermore, some children with cerebral palsy have specific defects of motor function (*apraxia*), of sensory function (*agnosia*), of the special senses (e.g. nerve deafness) or of speech and language (*aphasia, articulatory apraxia, dyslexia*—see Chapter 9); these can give a false impression of mental defect if clinical appraisal is superficial or limited. Thus specific defects of speech and other language functions are sometimes misdiagnosed as mental deficiency. However, if there is a discrepancy between basic intelligence and language function due to defects predominantly in the sphere of speech and language, then attempts should be made to compensate for the specific disorder by special methods of individual training either of the defective function or of the unaffected functions. It is very important that these children, as well as those with specific non-language disorders (as above), are recognised and educated appropriately; although requiring patient individual training, many can be helped considerably.

In some cases, motor disorders can be alleviated by surgical methods so helping these children to lead useful lives, but the prognosis will be poor if there are severe intellectual and motor deficits.

INFANTILE HEMIPLEGIA

Infantile hemiplegia can be present from birth (*congenital hemiplegia*) when it may be due to a cystic deformity of one cerebral hemisphere (*porencephaly*) or to infarction of the brain occurring *in utero*. More commonly it develops acutely in infancy or early childhood, often during the course of an acute infection such as whooping cough or following a 'febrile convulsion'. Probably the most common cause is cerebral infarction from arterial or venous occlusion, resulting in scarring and atrophy of the cerebral hemisphere with localised dilatation of the lateral ventricle.

The affected arm is severely paralysed, finger and hand movements being abolished and the hand and forearm assume a typically flexed posture lying across the front of the chest. The leg, though spastic with exaggerated tendon reflexes and an extensor plantar response, is less severely affected and all patients are eventually able to walk, often with surprisingly little difficulty.

Infantile hemiplegia is rarely bilateral; it can then be distinguished from a spastic diplegia due to cerebral palsy (Little's disease) by the fact that an infantile hemiplegia the upper limbs are more severely affected than the lower.

If the dominant hemisphere is involved after speech has developed, aphasia results; the earlier the age of the child the more complete and rapid is the recovery of speech function. If the dominant hemisphere is involved before speech is acquired, the development of speech may be delayed, but then speech function may become established in the opposite hemisphere.

Residual neurological deficits can be of all grades of severity, but are sometimes only trivial. In the more severe cases, epilepsy is a common complication as the scar in the affected hemisphere acts as an irritative focus. In those cases in which epileptic seizures are frequent and severe, brain damage is marked and intellectual impairment and behaviour disorders are common.

Further Reading

CARTER C.O. (1962) *Human Heredity.* Penguin Books, Harmondsworth.
LORING J. (ed.) (1968) *Assessment of the Cerebral Palsied Child for Education.* Heinemann Medical for Spastics Society, London.
MECHAM M.J., BERKO M.J. & BERKO F.G. (1960) *Speech Therapy in Cerebral Palsy.* C.C. Thomas, Springfield, Illinois.
PHAROAH P.O.D. (1981) Epidemiology of cerebral palsy: a review. *J. Roy. Soc. Med.* **74**, 516–20.
ROBERTS J.A.F. (1959) *An Introduction to Medical Genetics,* 2e. University Press, Oxford.

CHAPTER 16
INFECTIONS

Infections are the result of invasion of the body by microorganisms such as bacteria and viruses. These organisms vary in virulence (i.e. their capacity to spread and cause disease).

The factors which determine the result of an infection are the resistance or susceptibility of the host tissues (a high standard of general health and well-being will tend to improve resistance to infection), the virulence of the infecting organism and the sensitivity of the organism to treatment.

Bacteria are microscopic organisms which are universally disseminated. Each organism consists of one cell which has the capacity to multiply but only some produce disease (i.e. are pathogenic). Bacteria have various shapes, e.g. round (cocci), rod shaped (bacilli), but a high-power microscope is necessary to see these.

Viruses are also unicellular organisms but are smaller than bacteria. Infections due to viruses include the common cold, influenza, measles, poliomyelitis, small pox and chicken pox, herpes simplex and zoster. Viruses may infect the nervous system and cause meningitis or encephalitis (inflammation of the meninges or brain). Encephalitis may be diffuse and involve large areas of the brain, or be localised and result in abscess formation. The herpes simplex virus causes a very severe form of encephalitis, the maximum inflammation frequently involving the temporal lobes.

Inflammation

Tissues which become infected with an organism produce an inflammatory reaction, i.e. there is redness and swelling due to increase of the local blood supply (vasodilatation) with seepage of fluid and white blood cells (leucocytes and macrophages). Necrosis in the centre of the inflamed area may lead to pus formation and a surrounding capsule is formed by fibrous tissue. The pus-filled cavity increases in size and at the point of least resistance comes to the surface, where it may burst spontaneously, or require surgical evacuation of the pus. Provided that the infection is overcome by virtue of the resistance of the tissues and treatment with appropriate antibiotics, the inflammatory reaction will subside.

Abscess

An abscess is a localised pocket of infection containing pus (e.g. a boil is an abscess in the skin). In some parts of the body, if the pus cannot be evacuated, the abscess increases in size and penetrates deeply to cause increasing damage by compression.

A cerebral abscess is the result of an infection which reaches the brain either by direct spread from the middle ear (otitis media), or sinuses (sinusitis), or via the blood stream, e.g. from the lungs (pneumonia or pulmonary abscess). The cerebral abscess acts as an intracranial space-occupying lesion producing symptoms and signs of raised intracranial pressure, viz. headache, vomiting and papilloedema. Local effects are determined by its situation (e.g. it may cause focal epilepsy or neurological signs, including dysphasia if the speech area is involved).

Otitis media and mastoiditis

Infection of the middle ear may penetrate the petrous bone spreading anteriorly into the middle cranial fossa to involve the temporal lobe, or posteriorly into the posterior fossa to involve the adjacent cerebellar hemisphere. Abscesses can form in other parts of the brain, even on the side opposite to the infected ear, and may be multiple, indicating that the spread has been via the blood stream.

Local meningeal reaction or rupture of an intracerebral abscess leads to meningitis. Other complications from otitis media include lateral sinus thrombosis and cortical thrombo-phlebitis. The organisms that cause these infections are most commonly the staphylococcus, *Bacterium coli*, *Haemophilus influenzae* and proteus.

Meningitis

Inflammation of the meninges usually results from spread of a local infection or is a complication of a systemic infection, frequently viral. Bacterial meningitis in adults may be due to the meningococcus or pneumococcus and in children to *Haemophilus influenzae*, although any of the bacteria already mentioned may be responsible. Meningococcal meningitis (cerebro-spinal or 'spotted fever') occurs in epidemic form and, before the discovery of sulphonamides and antibiotics, was often fatal, but nowadays it is more amenable to treatment. It was called 'spotted-fever' because in fulminating cases, purpura (minute haemorrhagic spots) developed in the skin. Haemorrhage occasionally occurred in the adrenal glands causing death from adrenal failure.

Many of the complications of meningitis are the result of inflammatory exudate forming mainly at the base of the brain, so damaging the cranial nerves. Involvement of the 8th cranial (auditory) nerves, causing deafness, is most frequent, but damage to this nerve can also result from the toxic effects of streptomycin (one of the antibiotics used in the treatment of tuberculosis).

Tuberculosis

Infection with the tubercle bacillus (TB) most commonly involves the lungs (pulmonary tuberculosis). All forms of tuberculosis including tuberculous meningitis are now relatively rare in England but still common in Asia. Tuberculous abscesses more often occur in the cerebellar than cerebral hemispheres and are complications of tuberculosis of tissues elsewhere (e.g. the lungs), the infecting organisms (tubercle bacilli) being carried to the brain via the blood stream. As the tuberculous abscess enlarges, raised intracranial pressure develops. Alternatively a chronic granuloma (tuberculoma) is formed and may exist in the brain for months or even years without causing symptoms. It may become inactive and calcified showing up on X-rays of the skull as a rounded irregular calcified mass.

Syphilis

This is one of the venereal diseases which may produce local genital symptoms when contracted, and then remain latent to produce manifestations of involvement of the nervous system (neurosyphilis) many years later. There is also a congenital form of the disease due to transmission to the fetus by an infected mother. The spirochaete which causes syphilis, *Treponema pallidum*, is a corkscrew shaped microorganism, which invades the tissues to cause the specific inflammatory reaction of the disease. Neurosyphilis is now relatively rare, but the classical types are still recognised.

General paralysis of the insane (GPI)

GPI develops after a latent period following the acute infection, sometimes as long as 10–20 years later. The disease affects the cerebral hemispheres causing generalised atrophy, particularly of the cortex. The mental, intellectual and personality deterioration (*dementia*) is progressive unless early treatment with penicillin is given. There are generalised tremors, involving particularly the hands, lips and tongue. The tremor of the hands is usually fine and rapid, but the tremor of the tongue is sometimes coarse with backwards and forwards movements, aptly described as 'trombone tremor'. Bilateral pyramidal signs with increased tendon reflexes, clonus and extensor plantar responses are often present. There is a characteristic type of dysarthria which may be due to a combination of factors, viz. the tremor of the tongue, pseudobulbar palsy (due to bilateral upper motor neurone involvement), and cortical atrophy affecting the motor part of the speech area.

In all forms of neurosyphilis, pupillary abnormalities are frequently seen. The most characteristic is the *Argyll Robertson pupil*, which is small and irregular in outline; it does not react to light but does to accommodation. (Argyll Robertson was an Edinburgh ophthalmologist who first described these abnormalities.)

Tabes dorsalis

The clinical picture is due to involvement of the posterior horns of the spinal cord, the posterior root ganglia of the spinal nerves and the sensory components of the cranial nerves. The main effects of tabes, therefore, are on the sensory system, depending upon the distribution of the segments affected. Involvement of the posterior nerve roots and ganglia often results in severe pain which is typically shooting or lancinating in character (lightning pains) causing sudden horizontally or vertically directed stabs, usually affecting the legs. Various visceral crises with bouts of severe pain may involve, for example, the bladder, stomach or larynx.

Loss of sensation occurs in various parts of the body, particularly the legs, ulnar aspects of the forearms and hands, over the chest and on the face and nose. Loss of superficial pain sensation is tested with a pin and, instead of the pinprick, the patient feels only a blunt touch. There is loss of deep pain sensation which is tested by squeezing the muscles and tendons (e.g. the tendo-Achilles) which are normally pain-sensitive. Loss of temperature sensation results in inability to differentiate between hot and cold and patients may sustain burns without feeling pain. The sensory fibres conveying pain and temperature sensations cross to the opposite side of the spinal cord and ascend in the lateral spinothalamic tracts. The posterior roots also convey the senses of position and vibration, which are conveyed up the spinal cord by the fibres of the posterior columns. Because these are affected in patients with *tabes dorsalis* (the name literally means wasting of the dorsal columns), there is loss of position and vibration sense in the limbs. The position of various parts of the body can be checked visually, so the patient can compensate for loss of the sense of position, but there will be unsteadiness with a tendency to fall in the dark or with the eyes closed (e.g. when washing the face). Loss of position sense can be tested by asking the patient to stand up straight with the feet together; with the eyes open, balance is maintained but on closing the eyes, the patient sways and may fall due to loss of position sense in the feet and legs (Romberg's sign).

Because of interference with sensation to the skin, trophic changes may occur leading to ulceration which is often indolent and chronic. Interference with the sensation of joints leads to a painless form of arthropathy with gross deformities (Charcot's joints).

As a result of the loss of sensation from the bladder the patient may fail to appreciate when the bladder is full so that there is retention of urine, or overflow incontinence with an atonic bladder.

The loss of sensation also interferes with the reflex arc, so that the tendon reflexes in the limbs are reduced or absent.

Speech is not as a rule affected in tabes, except in cases having combined features of both tabes and GPI, which is then called *taboparesis.*

Meningovascular syphilis

As the name implies, the blood vessels and meninges are particularly involved. The meninges become inflamed and thickened due to a low grade meningitis in which headache is a marked feature. Thickening of the meninges at the base of the brain can also cause cranial nerve palsies. The lumen of the blood vessels, particularly those penetrating the meninges and supplying the surfaces of the brain, becomes narrowed and obliterated. Local areas of ischaemia result and cause focal epilepsy and neurological signs; according to the part involved, aphasia, monoplegia or hemiplegia, homonymous hemianopia or hemianaesthesia may develop.

Gumma

This is a mass of granulomatous tissue due to syphilis and can occur in almost any part of the body, including the brain. An intracerebral gumma is exceedingly rare but acts as a space-occupying lesion causing raised intracranial pressure with focal neurological deficits depending upon its situation.

The *differential diagnosis* of neurosyphilis includes many disorders of the nervous system which it can resemble. Fortunately laboratory tests of the serum and CSF are of great diagnostic value. Of these, the Wassermann Reaction (WR) is widely used, and is positive both in the serum and CSF in most patients with active neurosyphilis. More refined tests have now been developed, including the treponemal immobilisation (TPI) and fluorescent treponemal absorption (FTA) tests. In some cases the WR becomes negative after treatment with penicillin, but the TPI and FTA usually remain positive and so give additional evidence of previous spirochaetal infection.

All forms of neurosyphilis are now rare, as the acute venereal infection can be effectively treated with penicillin and other antibiotics. Penicillin is the best prophylactic and curative treatment of neurosyphilis, and previous methods using malaria, arsenic and bismuth preparations have been superseded.

Poliomyelitis

This is an infection of the anterior horn cells of the spinal cord and motor nuclei of the cranial nerves in the brain stem by the poliomyelitis virus. The acute stage lasts a few days with symptoms of a systemic illness, meningitis and sometimes encephalitis. If enough anterior horn cells in the spinal cord are involved paralysis of lower motor neurone type occurs, typically in a patchy distribution and, if the motor nuclei in the brain stem are affected, bulbar palsy occurs with dysarthria, dysphonia and dysphagia (see Chapter 7).

Bulbar palsy and respiratory paralysis may necessitate artificial respiration, either with a tank type of respirator or tracheostomy with a pump respirator (intermittent positive pressure respirator— IPPR). Not all cases develop paralysis but, in those that do, recovery can take place provided that sufficient anterior horn cells or motor nuclei remain undamaged. Dead neurones cannot be replaced but probably more than half the number of functioning cells have to be damaged before any clinical weakness results. After the acute stage of the illness, further recovery of function is possible because certain muscles are capable of retraining and hypertrophy to compensate for those affected.

The serious epidemics that used to occur can be prevented by vaccination so that acute poliomyelitis is now a rarity.

Further Reading

BRAIN W.R. & WALTON J. (1976) *Diseases of the Nervous System*, 8e. University Press, Oxford.

CHAPTER 17
VASCULAR DISORDERS

Blood supply of the brain

Four arteries in the neck carry the blood supply to the brain, namely the internal carotid and vertebral arteries on each side. The internal carotid arteries pass through the foramen lacerum at the base of the skull to follow a tortuous intracranial course (the carotid syphon). Above this each gives off the ophthalmic artery and then terminates by dividing into anterior and middle cerebral arteries. The vertebral arteries pass up through the vertebral canals in the transverse processes of the cervical vertebrae, coil around the arch of the atlas on each side and pass through the foramen magnum, above which they join to form the basilar artery; this artery ascends in the midline along the anterior aspect of the brain stem to which it gives off paired branches. At the upper level of the mid-brain the basilar artery terminates by dividing into the two posterior cerebral arteries. *The circle of Willis* (see Fig. 8) is completed by the posterior communicating arteries, which join the posterior cerebral to the internal carotid arteries and by the anterior communicating artery which joins the right and left anterior cerebral arteries.

STROKES

A stroke is an acute distrubance of brain function of vascular origin causing disability lasting more than 24 hours, or death. The three main causes are:
1 Haemorrhage.
2 Infarction.
3 Transient ischaemic attacks ('little strokes').

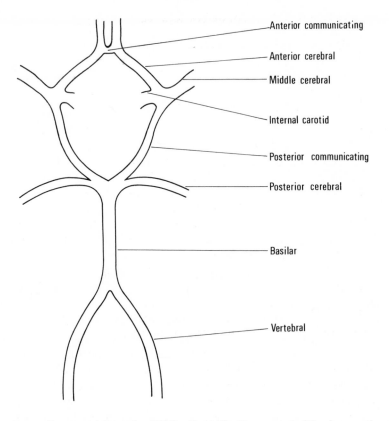

Anterior communicating

Anterior cerebral

Middle cerebral

Internal carotid

Posterior communicating

Posterior cerebral

Basilar

Vertebral

Fig. 8 Diagram of the circle of Willis. (From *The Management of Cerebrovascular Disease* 3e, by J. Marshall (1976). Churchill, London.)

Haemorrhage

Haemorrhage results from rupture of the wall of a blood vessel so that blood escapes from the circulation, either into the subarachnoid space (subarachnoid haemorrhage), the substance of the brain (intracerebral or intracerebellar) or into the ventricle (intraventricular); the blood may clot forming a haematoma.

Intracranial haemorrhage usually causes sudden headache, often with loss of consciousness. Within a few minutes, there are usually signs of meningeal irritation due to blood in the subarachnoid space, e.g. photophobia (dislike of light) and neck stiffness, which disappear if coma supervenes.

The commonest causes of intracranial haemorrhage are:

1 Atheroma and arteriosclerosis, with hypertension.
2 Aneurysm and angioma.
3 Bleeding diseases.
4 Trauma.

1 *Atheroma and arteriosclerosis*

The three layers of a vessel wall are (a) the *intima* which is the inner endothelial lining, (b) the *media* or muscular and elastic layer, and (c) the *adventitia* which is the connective tissue surrounding the blood vessel. Atheroma is the name given to the change in the arteries due to deposition of plaques of cholesterol in the intima. It usually affects the smaller and medium sized arteries and causes narrowing of the lumen. Arteriosclerosis occurs when the elastic tissue degenerates, the wall of the artery becomes thickened, irregular and tortuous, and microaneurysms may form on the capillaries. High blood pressure (which is commonly associated with degenerative arterial disease) will further aggravate the liability of the vessel wall to rupture, resulting in haemorrhage.

2 *Aneurysm*

This is a dilation of the artery, usually at a point of bifurcation, due to congenital weakness in the media. Most aneurysms are found on the main arteries of the *circle of Willis*, approximately 30% arising from the anterior group (i.e. the anterior cerebral and anterior communicating arteries), 30% directly from the internal carotid artery, usually at the level of the junction with the posterior communicating artery and 30% from the middle cerebral arteries. The remaining 10% are situated on the various other intracranial arteries (i.e. vertebral and basilar or their branches, or on the peripheral branches of the cerebral arteries).

The wall of an aneurysm is more liable to rupture as the patient gets older, when atheromatous changes become superimposed and hypertension develops. The seriousness of rupture of an intracranial aneurysm is evidenced by the fact that about 50% of patients die within four weeks and few survive more than two or three haemorrhages.

Another complication occurs if the sac of the aneurysm enlarges and compresses the neighbouring structures; for example, compression of the third cranial (oculo-motor) nerve by an aneurysm of the internal carotid artery at its junction with the posterior communicating artery causes an oculo-motor palsy, viz. ptosis, dilated pupil and paralysis of the external ocular muscles (excluding the superior oblique and lateral rectus muscles).

3 Angioma

An angioma is a congenital malformation consisting of a mass of abnormal blood vessels. It may be situated within the substance of one cerebral hemisphere or the brain stem, or superficially on the surface, sometimes extending deeply into the cerebral hemisphere in the shape of a wedge. The size varies from minute angiomas visible only with a microscope to extremely large ones involving almost the whole of one hemisphere; they are supplied by some or all of the main arteries of the circle of Willis. Instead of blood taking its normal time and course through the capillaries of the brain, these congenital anomalies form large arterio-venous communications or shunts which tend to deprive the underlying area of the brain of its normal blood supply. The vessels making up the angioma are abnormally thin and liable to rupture so that subarachnoid or intracerebral haemorrhages are common complications. Rupture of an angioma tends to occur at an earlier age than with an aneurysm and is less commonly fatal so that there may be a history of several haemorrhages.

Other complications of angioma are epilepsy and persistent neurological deficits such as dysphasia, depending on which part of the brain is involved.

4 Bleeding diseases

Subarachnoid and intracerebral haemorrhages, often minute but multiple, can result from haemorrhagic diseases in which there is some general disorder of the clotting mechanism of the blood (e.g. when there is a deficiency of platelets as in thrombocytopenia and some cases of leukaemia). Intracranial haemorrhage may also occur as a complication of anticoagulant therapy.

5   *Trauma*

Head injuries may cause haemorrhage or contusion in the substance of the brain, sometimes with bleeding into the subarachnoid space (traumatic subarachnoid haemorrhage). Bleeding may also occur into the extradural or subdural spaces forming localised clots (extradural or subdural haematoma); the resultant rise in intracranial pressure can cause severe, even fatal, complications because of compression and distortion of the cerebral hemispheres or brain stem. In any severe head injury with intracranial haemorrhage there may be a fracture of the skull and concussion. Concussion is the 'knock-out' of brain function that follows a head injury, i.e. the immediate loss of consciousness, confusion and amnesia that are reversible and not due to any *visible* brain damage which may or may not coexist (see Chapter 19).

Investigations

Lumbar puncture in subarachnoid haemorrhage reveals uniformly blood-stained CSF instead of the normally clear and colourless fluid. If the specimen is centrifuged or allowed to stand, the supernatant fluid has a yellow tinge (*xanthochromia*).

X-rays of the skull may show a fracture, or displacement of the calcified pineal gland, for example, by an intracranial haematoma. (The pineal gland appears calcified in the skull X-rays of about 50% of normal people and should be in the midline.) Echoencephalography (using an ultrasonoscope) may also indicate shift of midline structures and scanning techniques using radioactive isotopes may demonstrate the position and size of lesions. The introduction of the CT scanner (using an X-ray technique called computerised tomography) has changed the mode of investigation of strokes so that lumbar puncture, echoencephalography and isotope scanning are rarely used.

The CT scanner indicates the position and often the pathological nature of intracranial lesions and is capable of distinguishing an intracerebral haemorrhage from an infarct. In order to ascertain the state of the blood vessels, angiography (a radiological technique involving the injection of a radiopaque fluid into either of the carotid or vertebral arteries in the neck) is necessary, particularly when surgical intervention is being considered. The radiopaque fluid is carried with the circulating blood into the intracranial blood vessels which are then revealed by X-rays. An intracranial haematoma (extradural, subdural or intracerebral) is demonstrated by displacement of the blood vessels (e.g. instead of the anterior cerebral artery lying almost in the midline, it may be displaced towards the opposite side); an aneurysm is shown as a small diverticulum on an artery; an angioma as a tangle of knotted vessels on the surface of, and perhaps extending deeply into, one cerebral hemisphere; atheroma and arteriosclerosis are revealed by narrowing, irregularity and tortuosity of the arteries.

Treatment

Intracranial haematoma can be removed surgically. If an aneurysm is found, the management depends on its exact situation since many are now accessible to surgery by ligation or clipping of the neck or base of the aneurysm close to its junction with the wall of the artery. This prevents any future rupture as the aneurysmal sac is excluded from the circulation. An alternative method is to wrap a piece of muscle or synthetic material around the fundus of the sac to strengthen the wall and prevent any recurrent rupture. Yet another method of treatment is to reduce the pressure in the arteries leading to the aneurysm by ligation of the common carotid artery in the neck. When the patient is hypertensive, the blood pressure can be effectively lowered by hypotensive drugs.

Infarction

Infarction is death of tissue (necrosis) due to impairment of the blood supply (ischaemia). If the cells of the nervous system (neurones) are deprived of their blood supply for more than a few minutes, they cannot survive and there will be an area of cerebral infarction. The extent of the infarct and the resultant neurological deficits will depend not only on which vessel is obstructed but also on the capacity of neighbouring arteries to supplement the deficient blood supply, (i.e. develop a *collateral circulation*).

The two main causes of prolonged or severe ischaemia sufficient to produce infarction are thrombosis and embolism.

1   *Thrombosis*

Intravascular clot formation (thrombosis) is commonly due to atheroma with slowing of the blood flow. The clot causing the obstruction may develop either in the intra- or extracranial parts of the carotid and vertebral arteries; this is liable to result in cerebral infarction particularly if the intracranial vessels are arteriosclerotic, which reduces the capacity to form a collateral circulation.

Investigations

The CT scan shows a cerebral infarct as an area of reduced density. The cerebrospinal fluid is nearly always clear (i.e. not obviously blood-stained) and carotid arteriography may show the point of obstruction in the affected artery. At least 20% of strokes are due to occlusion of the extracranial part of the internal carotid artery in the neck just above the bifurcation of the common carotid artery.

Treatment

In some cases it may be possible to remove the thrombus surgically, if it is near the origin of the internal carotid artery in the neck and if the block is not complete. This may be justified if serious cerebral deficit has not already developed, and the long-term results of such procedures are usually good. In recent years, an operation has been developed to increase the blood flow to the brain. This is done by joining (anastomosing) a branch of the external carotid artery (usually the superficial temporal) with a distal branch of the internal carotid artery (usually the middle cerebral); this serves to bypass the block in the internal carotid artery.

Anticoagulant therapy is contra-indicated in acute cerebral infarction due to thrombosis because of the danger of bleeding into the infarcted brain tissue. Severe hypertension can be treated with hypotensive drugs but care must be taken not to reduce the blood pressure below a certain level as this may further impair the cerebral circulation and interfere with recovery.

2   *Embolism*

An embolus is a fragment of clot or other substance (e.g. fat, air, aggregations of platelets, fibrin or cholesterol) which is carried in the circulation from one part of the body and obstructs a blood vessel elsewhere. Embolism is liable to occur in various heart diseases, for example when the auricles are not contracting properly (auricular fibrillation) so that the blood in the auricles becomes stagnant and forms clots. Fragments break off, pass through the auricular–ventricular valves (mitral or tricuspid) to be expelled via the main arteries and carried in the circulation, eventually obstructing smaller blood vessels such as the cerebral arteries supplying the brain. If the obstruction is not relieved (e.g. by further fragmentation or absorption of the embolus) and if the collateral circulation is inadequate, the area of brain involved will become infarcted. Embolism also occurs in myocardial disease secondary to coronary thrombosis, i.e. a clot in the coronary arteries supplying the heart, so that there is infarction of the heart muscle (*myocardial infarction*). This may involve the inner lining of the heart (*endocardium*) with formation of a clot on the endocardial surface. If this fragments, emboli may then be carried via the aorta into any of the main arteries in the body and cerebral embolism may result.

Cerebral embolism presents with an extremely sudden disturbance of function, the resulting signs depending upon which part of the brain is rendered ischaemic. Dysphasia and hemiplegia due to a cerebral embolus will have an acute onset followed by improvement. Although recovery in some cases is slow and incomplete, in others there is no loss of consciousness and the prognosis is excellent. Specific medical or surgical treatment is directed to the underlying cause of the clot formation and anticoagulant therapy is used in some cases.

TRANSIENT ISCHAEMIC ATTACKS

Occlusion of blood vessels by thrombosis or embolism is not necessarily complete and the ischaemia may be insufficient to cause infarction. A transient ischaemic attack (TIA) is an acute disturbance of brain or retinal function due to ischaemia (impairment of the blood supply) causing disability which lasts less than 24 hours. Most TIAs last less than 6 hours, many are fleeting and recur and those affecting the brain are sometimes referred to as 'little strokes'.

Repeated TIAs may be due to microembolism by atheromatous material and platelet–fibrin aggregates. A common site of origin of these microemboli is from an atheromatous plaque (patch of atheroma) on the internal carotid artery just above the bifurcation of the common carotid artery in the neck. TIAs affecting the cerebral hemispheres, retina or brain stem are commonly encountered in arteriosclerotic patients with narrowing (stenosis) of the internal carotid or vertebral arteries. If this can be confirmed by arteriography and if the narrowed segment is localised in an accessible situation in a relatively young patient, it may be treated surgically. Carotid endarterectomy or reconstruction is highly successful in preventing both recurrent attacks and subsequent major strokes. Anticoagulant therapy may also be effective in some cases, and more recent studies suggest that treatment with aspirin and other drugs which reduce the aggregation of platelets can stop the attacks and prevent strokes.

The vertebral arteries are vulnerable to obstruction in the vertebral canal of the cervical spine and in their upper part as they curve round the transverse processes of the atlas. Excessive or prolonged movements of the head and neck can interfere with the circulation via the vertebral arteries, particularly when these are arteriosclerotic. In middle aged and elderly subjects, there is often cervical spondylosis, i.e. degeneration of the cervical spine with narrowing of the disc spaces, the small joints becoming deformed with bony irregularities (*osteophytes*). These may impinge on the vertebral arteries and impede the circulation especially when the head is turned or the neck extended.

Transient ischaemic attacks affecting the brain stem are referred to as 'vertebro–basilar insufficiency'. The symptoms are due to the disturbances of brain stem function resulting from involvement of cranial nerve nuclei, e.g. defects of eye movements and diplopia (3rd, 4th and 6th), sensory loss on the face (5th), facial weakness (7th), tinnitus, deafness, vertigo and nystagmus (8th), loss of palatal sensation (9th), palatal weakness, dysphagia, dysphonia and dysarthria (10th, 11th and 12th). Involvement of the sympathetic fibres in the brain stem will cause Horner's syndrome (partial ptosis, constriction of the pupil, and loss of sweating on the forehead of the affected side). In addition there may be incoordination and ataxia of the limbs, nystagmus and ataxic dysarthria from ischaemia of the cerebellum and its connections.

As mentioned previously, if the ischaemia lasts longer than the critical period, infarction will result and the same neurological deficits are prolonged or permanent. Transient ischaemic episodes recurring repeatedly may thus herald the onset of a major stroke. Sometimes it is possible to relieve these transient attacks, for example by restriction of neck movements (using a collar).

Conditions causing fall in cardiac output and blood pressure also produce transient cerebral ischaemia and this is the mechanism of fainting (*syncope*). The fall in blood pressure results in defective blood supply to the brain stem and cerebral hemispheres producing the symptoms of faintness, dizziness, blurred vision and nausea, etc., leading to loss of consciousness; the patient falls to the ground and this lowering of the head restores the blood supply to the brain so that recovery is rapid. There are many causes of syncope, e.g. vaso–vagal attacks, cough syncope, hypotension and cardiac disorders such as heart block (*Stokes-Adams attacks*). Sometimes it is necessary to monitor the electrocardiogram to demonstrate that TIAs are related to a cardiac dysrhythmia.

Spasm of cerebral blood vessels (narrowing due to contraction of the muscle wall) is occasionally seen in arteriograms and at operation following subarachnoid haemorrhage. If the period of ischaemia is short, infarction does not occur and recovery follows when the spasm clears and the blood supply is restored. Spasm or vasoconstriction producing cerebral, retinal or brain stem ischaemia is also thought to account for the transient premonitory symptoms (e.g. visual, sensory and sometimes speech disturbances —see page 38) which occur in *migraine*, the headache being associated with the subsequent vasodilatation.

Further Reading

GANN R. (1978) *Stroke: a Bibliography.* Wessex Regional Library and Information Service, Southampton.
MARSHALL J. (1976) *The Management of Cerebrovascular Disease*, 3e. Blackwell Scientific Publications, Oxford.
ROSE F.C. & CAPILDEO R. (1981) *Stroke: the Facts.* University Press, Oxford.
ROSE F.C. & GAWEL M. (1980) *Migraine: the Facts.* University Press, Oxford.

CHAPTER 18
TUMOURS

Pathology

Tumours are abnormal growths (neoplasms), which may be either primary or secondary. A primary tumour consists of cells derived from those of the tissue in which it develops. These cells proliferate and the resulting tumour may be benign or malignant.

A *benign* tumour grows slowly, and does not infiltrate, invade locally or spread to other parts of the body. It remains confined to the structure of origin, is often encapsulated and its main effects are due to compression of the surrounding tissues.

A *malignant* tumour (cancer) infiltrates the tissues in which it develops and invades neighbouring structures; many malignant tumours metastasise (i.e. spread to other parts of the body), because the malignant cells of the primary growth infiltrate into the lymphatic or blood vessels and are then transported to organs elsewhere. These cells then form secondary tumours or deposits (metastases) which continue to grow in the same way. Secondary tumours which result from the spread of primary malignant tumours consist of cells similar to those of the primary tumour.

Tumour cells as seen under a microscope have characteristic shapes and patterns resembling the cells of the tissues from which they arise. The most malignant tumours consist of mainly primitive and poorly differentiated cells which tend to proliferate rapidly. Cell multiplication takes place by the process of division called 'mitosis' and the demonstration under the microscope of dividing cells (i.e. cells undergoing mitosis) usually indicates that the tumour is malignant.

The names given to tumours (whether benign or malignant) frequently end in the suffix '-oma' (e.g. meningioma, astrocytoma) the first part of the name indicating the structure or type of cells from which the tumour originates. The suffix '-blastoma' implies that the tumour is composed of blast or primitive cells which are usually highly malignant. Some malignant tumours are referred to as carci-

167

noma, the commonest being carcinoma of the bronchus in males, and carcinoma of the breast in females, but primary malignant tumours can originate in almost any structure of the body and if they metastasise via the blood stream, their secondary deposits may develop in various sites, including the brain (see page 178).

Clinical manifestations

The clinical manifestations of intracranial tumours include:

1 Local symptoms and signs, dependent on the site of the tumour and on its rate of growth.
2 Focal or generalised epileptic attacks, depending on whether there is involvement of one or both cerebral hemispheres (see Chapter 14).
3 The effects of raised intracranial pressure (i.e. headache, vomiting, papilloedema and sometimes false localising signs).

These may occur singly or in any combination.

Raised intracranial pressure

As the skull—except in childhood (see below)—is a rigid structure, the total volume of the cranial cavity is fixed, the normal contents being the brain, blood and cerebrospinal fluid (CSF). The proportion of these varies with physiological changes but the intracranial pressure is maintained within a limited range. As an intracranial tumour enlarges, it is liable to cause an increase in intracranial pressure, resulting from (a) the mass effect of the tumour (sometimes with secondary haemorrhage or venous congestion), (b) the development of brain oedema (swelling) and (c) obstruction to the circulation of CSF.

The mechanical effects of displacement of the brain by a supratentorial space-occupying lesion include herniation of the lower medial part of the temporal lobe (the uncus) through the opening of the tentorium (tentorial herniation) so compressing or displacing the brain stem downwards and stretching the cranial nerves on the affected side (especially the 3rd and 6th). The effects of this are the result of damage to structures remote from the tumour: 'false localising signs'. A posterior fossa mass (i.e. infratentorial) may compress or displace the brain stem upwards, and the cerebellar tonsils downwards through the foramen magnum causing a cerebellar pressure cone, which in turn compresses the medulla.

The headache of raised intracranial pressure is typically worse on waking, aggravated by coughing, straining and stooping, and is often accompanied by vomiting. *Papilloedema* is the term describing swelling of the optic nerve head (the papilla) as seen with an ophthalmoscope. This is usually associated with venous engorgement and reflects the high intracranial pressure transmitted along the sheath of the optic nerve which is continuous with the meninges. Initially vision is not affected but if the raised intracranial pressure is not relieved and the papilloedema increases, then the optic nerve will be damaged, retinal haemorrhages develop and vision fails. Unrelieved, the effect on the brain stem will lead to progressive impairment of consciousness, interference with the vital mechanisms in the medulla and death.

Longstanding increase in the intracranial pressure can be detected sometimes by X-rays showing thinning of certain parts of the skull bones, particularly around the pituitary fossa (e.g. erosion of the posterior clinoid processes). In children, the sutures of the bones of the skull vault do not fuse completely until about the age of 10 and a rise in intracranial pressure before that can cause separation of the sutures. The head may then enlarge and the skull bones become thinned, leading to an actual increase in the circumference of the skull and a 'cracked pot' note on percussion. Obstruction to the exit of CSF from the 4th ventricle in the brain stem will cause dilatation of the 3rd ventricle and the lateral ventricles in the cerebral hemispheres which can also be shown radiologically (e.g. with the CT scan).

TYPES OF INTRACRANIAL TUMOURS

Primary intracranial tumours originate from the structures within the skull. The commonest are:

1   Gliomas—malignant tumours of various types arising from the glial cells within the brain.
2   Meningioma—a benign tumour arising from the meninges.
3   Pituitary tumours—several types arising in the pituitary gland.

4   Other types—primary intracranial tumours growing from a variety of persistent embryonic tissues. These include pinealoma, craniopharyngioma, haemangioblastoma, epidermoid, dermoid, colloid cysts and chordoma.

5   Acoustic neuroma—a benign tumour (neurofibroma) arising from the sheath of the 8th cranial nerve.

Secondary intracranial tumours (i.e. intracranial metastases) will be described later (see page 178).

Most primary intracranial tumours grow either exclusively or most commonly in certain situations (e.g. some involve the cerebral hemispheres—i.e. above the tentorium—others involve the cerebellum and medulla in the posterior fossa—i.e. below the tentorium). It is helpful therefore to describe various pathological types according to their usual site of origin, as this determines to a large extent their clinical picture.

Glioma

Gliomas are the commonest primary malignant tumours of the brain and originate from the glial cells (i.e. astrocytes, oligodendrocytes and microglia) which form the connective tissue of the brain, and are named according to the microscopic appearances of their cells.

The commonest type of glioma is an *astrocytoma* which is derived from cells of the astrocyte type, are locally malignant and infiltrate the brain substance but do not metastasise outside the nervous system. The rate of growth and spread of astrocytomas vary and different grades of malignancy can be recognised microscopically. These grades are numbered 1–4, the most malignant being grade 4 which is called glioblastoma multiforme or spongioblastoma, and recognised by the presence of undifferentiated primitive cells frequently seen in mitosis. This type often presents with epilepsy, raised intracranial pressure, and focal neurological deficits. The more malignant gliomas form many abnormal blood vessels so that the tumour is very vascular. Haemorrhages are then liable to occur spontaneously or on biopsy (i.e. surgical removal of a small piece of tumour for diagnostic microscopic examination). There is progressive deterioration leading to death often within months from the onset of symptoms. On the other hand grade 1 astrocytoma can be very slow growing, the first indication of a cerebral lesion (e.g. an epileptic fit) occurring sometimes as long as 5, 10 or even 15 years before death. Gliomas of the corpus callosum may spread into both cerebral hemispheres and present with dementia.

Oligodendrogliomas are derived from the oligodendrocytes, and usually grow very slowly. Like the slow-growing astrocytomas, calcification often occurs in them and can be seen radiologically. Sometimes, large cysts form within an astrocytoma, fill up with fluid and cause raised intracranial pressure; these can be aspirated with relief of pressure symptoms.

The prognosis with gliomas is usually poor since infiltration of the brain substance prevents removal of all the tumour, which probably extends further than is obvious to the naked eye at operation. Complete removal and cure is occasionally achieved (e.g. if an astrocytoma grade 1 is diagnosed early while still confined to the anterior part of a frontal or temporal lobe which may be excised in toto). Although radiotherapy is given in some cases, the results are not very encouraging as these tumours are rarely radiosensitive.

Meningioma

This is a primary tumour of the meninges and can develop in the spinal canal as well as intracranially; it is more common in women.

Meningiomas are benign tumours (i.e. they grow relatively slowly, do not actively infiltrate the brain and do not metastasise). The local effects are due to direct compression or displacement of the brain in which they become embedded. Raised intracranial pressure eventually develops and, if not relieved, death will ensue. These tumours usually grow into spherical shaped or irregular, lobulated masses with a relatively small point of attachment where the tumour originated from the dura and their complete neurosurgical removal is often possible. Unfortunately this is not always the case as sometimes these tumours extend as a solid layer (*meningioma en plaque*). They may also produce thickening of the overlying bone (*hyperostosis*) and occasionally erode through the skull to form a palpable or visible swelling on the head. There is a predilection for certain sites and the symptoms and signs will vary with the structures involved.

Olfactory groove meningioma will compress or displace one or both olfactory nerves, and cause unilateral or bilateral loss of the sense of smell (*anosmia*). As it increases in size it may compress the optic nerve causing loss of vision with primary optic atrophy. Raised intracranial pressure may supervene with generalised headache, vomiting and papilloedema. The combination of unilateral optic atrophy due to compression of the optic nerve by the tumour with papilloedema of the other optic nerve due to raised intracranial pressure is known as the *Foster Kennedy* syndrome. Olfactory groove meningiomas also compress the frontal lobes of the cerebral hemispheres causing changes in personality, behaviour and mood, often with disinhibition and mental and intellectual deterioration. Sometimes the main feature is apathy, loss of drive and initiative, performance at work deteriorates with inefficiency and flagging of interest in hobbies or other activities. This is often combined with apparently total lack of concern or insight on the part of the patient, much to the anxiety of friends and relations.

Another sign of a tumour in this situation is a 'grasp' reflex (i.e. the hand grasps involuntarily or reflexly anything that touches the palm). This is a primitive reflex seen normally during the first few months of life in infants, who grasp a finger or other object placed across the palm and do not let go unless forced to do so. Another manifestation of frontal lobe lesions is loss of control of micturition, usually with incontinence.

Involvement of the motor area will lead to *contralateral* facial palsy (of upper motor neurone type), weakness of the hand (*monoparesis*) and leg (*hemiparesis*). If the tumour is in the frontal lobe of the dominant cerebral hemisphere and impinges on Broca's area, this will cause dysphasia. Not infrequently frontal lobe tumours present with epileptic attacks, sometimes with *status epilepticus*.

Parasagittal or *convexity* meningioma originates from the falx near the sagittal sinus or the dura mater over the convexity of the cerebral hemispheres. Parasagittal meningioma may present with focal epilepsy starting in the opposite foot with transient motor or sensory disturbances which later become persistent and progressive. Involvement of the parietal lobe causes disturbance of sensation on the opposite side of the body (see page 13) and various types of apraxia and agnosia (see Chapter 3).

Sphenoidal ridge meningioma arises from the region of the greater or lesser wing of the sphenoid bone. The tumour enlarges in the middle fossa to compress the temporal lobe causing temporal lobe epilepsy (see Chapter 14). If the tumour is on the side of the dominant cerebral hemisphere, dysphasia develops. Involvement of the lower fibres of the optic radiation will produce contralateral homonymous upper quadrantic visual field defects, progressing to a complete homonymous hemianopia if the whole of the optic radiation becomes involved (see page 15).

Parasellar meningioma occurs around the pituitary fossa. The tumour presses on the optic nerve, chiasm or tract, causing the corresponding visual field defects and optic atrophy.

Tentorial meningioma arises from the tentorium cerebelli and grows either in a supratentorial direction compressing either one or both cerebral hemispheres, or downwards (infratentorially) into the posterior fossa compressing the cerebellum and brain stem. In the latter case there will be signs of cerebellar dysfunction, which may include dysarthria (see Chapter 7).

The diagnosis of meningioma can sometimes be suspected if the plain X-rays of the skull show a localised area of erosion or sclerosis of the bone overlying the tumour. A major advance in recent years is the development of the CT scan as meningiomas nearly always show on this and the picture of the tumour can be enhanced by contrast. Arteriography is also useful, although an 'invasive' investigation (see page 161); it usually reveals a meningioma which displaces and stretches arteries and veins, and typically shows a 'radiological blush' due to its vascularity (the blush resulting from filling of the tumour blood vessels with the radiopaque dye). The prognosis is usually very good after neurosurgical removal, which relieves the raised intracranial pressure; the focal neurological signs regress and may clear completely if the damage has not been too severe or longstanding. Epileptic attacks also cease unless there has been irreversible damage of the cerebral cortex by the tumour prior to removal. If the tumour has interfered with the blood supply to part of the brain, neurological disability may prove to be permanent. It is not always possible to remove the tumour completely so that, some time after the operation, signs recur due to regrowth of the remaining tumour. This occasionally takes on a more rapidly growing form with less differentiated cells (meningiosarcoma). Because of the danger of recurrence, radiotherapy may be advised postoperatively.

Dysphasia results from a meningioma pressing on the speech area, and dysarthria from a posterior fossa meningioma involving the brain stem or cerebellum. These speech disorders, like the other effects, will be progressive unless the tumour is removed. Post-operative speech therapy may help to enhance recovery of language function and compensate for residual defects. Various factors influence the prognosis for recovery of speech (see Chapter 5).

Pituitary tumours

The pituitary gland (often called the conductor of the endocrine orchestra because it secretes hormones which govern the other ductless glands) is situated at the base of the brain. Several types of tumour, depending on its main type of cell, may develop. The commonest are pituitary *adenomas* which are most frequently chromophobe, but eosinophil and basophil types also occur.

Craniopharyngioma is a tumour developing from embryonic remnants near the pituitary and has similar effects. The main clinical effects of pituitary tumours are:

1   Endocrine
    (a) Hypopituitarism—due to compression of the pituitary gland by the tumour interfering with production of one or more pituitary hormones, so causing secondary defects of gonadal (sex), adrenal or thyroid functions.
    (b) Hyperprolactinaemia—due to a prolactin secreting pituitary tumour, usually a chromophobe adenoma. In women this causes amenorrhaoea and infertility, and sometimes galactorrhoea, and in men—impotence.
    (c) Acromegaly—due to excessive production of growth hormone by the tumour cells.
    (d) Cushing's syndrome—due to excessive production of adreno-corticotrophic hormone (ACTH) by the tumour cells.

2   Compression of optic pathways
The optic chiasm lies anterior to and above the pituitary fossa and is particularly vulnerable to pressure from an expanding pituitary tumour. The characteristic visual field defect which results from chiasmal compression is bitemporal hemianopia (see Fig. 9) due to damage to the nasal crossing fibres of the optic nerves which convey images from the temporal halves of both visual fields. Neurosurgical treatment is indicated for relief of failing vision.

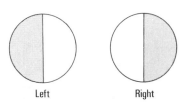

Left　　　　Right

Fig. 9　Bitemporal hemianopia.

3　The effects of suprasellar extension
Pituitary tumours can grow upwards out of the sella turcica and extend into the anterior or middle cranial fossae. This will compress the adjacent temporal or frontal areas of the cerebral hemispheres, causing focal epilepsy (e.g. with temporal lobe features) or motor deficits (e.g. facial weakness of upper motor neurone type). Dysphasia is a rare complication as the speech area lies on the lateral surface of the dominant cerebral hemisphere.

Pineal tumour

A pineal tumour is one involving the pineal body (a small gland situated in the posterior wall of the 3rd ventricle). These tumours, sometimes called pinealomas, may compress the 3rd ventricle and aqueduct and block the flow of CSF so causing obstructive hydro-cephalus (see Chapter 15). Other effects depend upon the main directions of growth of the tumour. There may be compression or invasion of the cerebral hemispheres or the tumour may extend downwards compressing the posterior aspect of the mid-brain at the level of the corpora quadrigemina. This interferes with con-jugate eye movements, typically causing defective upward gaze.

Pineal tumours as a rule are not accessible for neurosurgical re-moval, but radiotherapy is effective in some. The hydrocephalus can be treated surgically, by making a shunt so that the CSF can bypass the obstruction and be absorbed. One of the methods used involves inserting a Spitz-Holter valve; this is connected with a tube put into the lateral ventricle and a pumping device takes the CSF into the jugular vein in the neck.

Other rare tumours

Ependymoma. They are tumours derived from the ependymal cells which line the ventricles and are situated deeply in the substance of the brain. Other types which develop in the ventricles include *colloid cysts* and *papilloma* of the choroid plexus. Any of these can occur supratentorially in the 3rd or lateral ventricles, or infratentorially in the 4th ventricle.

Posterior fossa tumours

The main *primary* tumours of the cerebellum are:

1 Astrocytoma.
2 Haemangioblastoma.
3 Medulloblastoma.

Astrocytoma of the cerebellum

In children astrocytomas occur more frequently in the cerebellum than in the cerebral hemispheres. They are often cystic, slowly progressive and invade the cerebellum and brain stem. Occasionally they originate in and remain confined to the brain stem, particularly affecting the nuclei of the cranial nerves.

Haemangioblastoma

These are usually benign encapsulated tumours, composed mainly of blood vessel forming cells. Often cystic, they may contain large amounts of fluid with a relatively small tumour embedded in the wall (mural nodule). These tumours can often be removed completely.

Medulloblastoma

These occur almost invariably in children and are very malignant tumours of the brain stem and cerebellar vermis. They are locally invasive and extend deeply into the floor of the 4th ventricle. Being friable, fragments break off and circulate in the CSF, becoming attached to the surface of other parts of the neuraxis (e.g. the spinal cord). This type of spread is called 'seeding'. Medulloblastomas are initially radiosensitive but often recur so that the prognosis is poor.

Acoustic neuroma

Situated in the cerebello-pontine angle, an acoustic neuroma or neurofibroma is a benign primary tumour which grows from the sheath of the 8th cranial (acoustic) nerve. Very rarely they are bilateral and occasionally neurofibromas arise on the 5th cranial (trigeminal) nerve.

In a small percentage of cases (10–15%) acoustic neuroma may be associated with multiple neurofibromatosis (Von Recklinghausen's disease). In this condition, the tumours grow on the peripheral nerves in the skin and subcutaneous tissue; it is often associated with pigmented (café-au-lait) patches on the skin. Skeletal deformities can develop and tumours on the spinal nerve roots may compress the spinal cord.

An acoustic neuroma interferes with 8th nerve functions (auditory and vestibular) causing unilateral deafness, tinnitus and vertigo. The deafness is perceptive in type and progressive. Tinnitus is a hallucination of sound and the patient may be aware, for example, of a continuous hum or hiss in the affected ear. Vertigo is a hallucination of movement, usually rotatory, similar to the sensation experienced immediately after getting off a roundabout. If not detected and removed while still small, an acoustic neuroma will also cause the following:

1 Involvement of other cranial nerves, particularly the 7th and 5th, resulting in facial weakness and numbness, including loss of the corneal reflex, and loss of taste on the affected side.
2 Compression of the cerebellar hemisphere with incoordination of the arm and leg on the same side, nystagmus and dysarthria.
3 Compression of the brain stem producing pyramidal (UMN) signs.
4 Raised intracranial pressure—viz. headache, vomiting and papilloedema.

Although the tumour is benign and encapsulated, its situation is such that as it enlarges, it will compress and adhere to surrounding structures including the brain stem, and cause raised intracranial pressure which will be fatal if not relieved. Neurosurgery is therefore necessary as a lifesaving measure but, at this stage, when the tumour is large, the operation has a significant mortality and high morbidity. For example, the 7th cranial nerve, being in such close proximity to the 8th nerve during its course from the brain stem to the facial canal, is frequently compressed by the tumour and may have to be sacrificed during removal of the tumour. The facial palsy which ensues is disfiguring and initially may cause dysarthria; patients usually learn to compensate for this and pronounce words quite clearly by talking out of the unaffected side of the mouth. Plastic surgery can improve the cosmetic effect and faciohypoglossal nerve anastomosis provides reasonable function in the facial muscles, the unilateral paralysis and wasting of the tongue (resulting from division of the hypoglossal nerve) being relatively unimportant.

The dysarthria resulting from damage to the cerebellum or the lower cranial nerves often persists postoperatively and speech therapy is indicated to improve articulation. With involvement of the 10th cranial (vagus) nerve, nasal voice, dysphonia and dysphagia may occur but usually improve postoperatively.

As mentioned in Chapter 11, by investigating all cases of unilateral deafness, the early diagnosis of an acoustic neuroma is now possible using modern otological tests and CT scan. Microsurgical techniques enable the otologist and neurosurgeon, using the operating microscope, to remove the tumour while still only small, with negligible mortality and much less morbidity than before, and preservation of the facial nerve.

Intracranial metastases

Metastases are secondary deposits which result from spread of a primary malignant tumour, the commonest being from a carcinoma of the bronchus or breast (see page 168). Intracranial metastases may be deposited anywhere in the cerebral or cerebellar hemispheres, their localisation determining the symptoms and signs that they produce. They are usually multiple and not only enlarge progressively but also cause haemorrhages and oedema (swelling) within the brain with a rapid rise in intracranial pressure. An epileptic attack is sometimes the first indication of a cerebral metastasis. Occasionally there is only a single secondary deposit and sometimes symptoms and signs from this develop before any evidence of the primary tumour is detected, although this is unusual.

However, there have been rare cases of successful excision of a solitary metastasis, which on histological examination has revealed the nature of the previously unsuspected or undiscovered primary tumour, leading to its localisation and removal, and so effecting a cure. Unfortunately more often metastases are not only multiple (e.g. in the brain) but also scattered, involving the lymph glands and bones as well. These may be detected by CT scanning of the whole body, as well as of the head.

In a few cases the metastases from a primary malignant tumour develop on the meninges so that there are multiple meningeal deposits (carcinomatosis of the meninges) causing severe headaches and often random involvement of cranial nerves.

CHAPTER 19

TRAUMA

The type of speech disturbance resulting from head injury depends on the site and extent of the structural damage to the brain. Damage to the language area in the dominant cerebral hemisphere causes dysphasia, and damage to the brain stem or cerebellar connections causes dysarthria. Many head injuries are relatively minor and superficial and cause no obvious damage to the brain; even with a linear fracture of the vault of the skull, the brain may escape detectable damage. However, brain damage often occurs when there has been a fracture of the skull, particularly if bone fragments are depressed.

A violent blow or blunt injury delivered to the head, or the head hitting forcibly on a fixed surface, may or may not cut the scalp or fracture the skull, but the sudden acceleration or deceleration of the brain within the skull causes diffuse damage or extensive areas of focal damage determined by the force of the impact and by the shearing strains within the brain substance. If the injury causes a depressed fracture of the skull, the underlying cerebral cortex will suffer maximum damage, but there may also be 'contrecoup' or other more widespread effects.

With penetrating injuries (e.g. a high-velocity bullet) there is penetration of the dura mater with direct damage to the brain which may be localised or extensive; the neurological signs reflect the site, depth and extent of the brain damage. Depression of the inner table of the skull may have to be elevated surgically, and fragments of bone driven into the brain together with the penetrating missile itself may have to be removed.

Diffuse damage in its mildest form is reflected by *concussion* (i.e. 'the knockout' of brain function) as evidenced by loss of consciousness, confusion and amnesia following immediately on the head injury and due to brain damage which is not macroscopically visible. With severe injuries, in addition to concussion, there may also be shearing strains and tearing of nerve fibres as well as haemorrhages contributing to the disruption.

Head injuries do not necessarily cause concussion, so there may be no loss of awareness or loss of memory, but if there is brain damage from a closed (non-penetrating) head injury, the patient is usually unconscious for at least a short time. On regaining consciousness, there may be a further period of confusion or disorientation, and after recovery the patient does not remember events during part or all of this period from the moment of impact. This is *post-traumatic amnesia* and, as it may continue after consciousness appears to have been regained, calculation of its duration should include the total period of unconsciousness and/or amnesia from the moment of impact until continuous memory is restored.

After recovery from concussion it is often evident that there has also been loss of memory for a period of time leading up to and immediately preceding the impact; this is known as *retrograde amnesia*. This duration of unconsciousness following a head injury and of the posttraumatic amnesia are largely dependent on and related to the severity of the head injury and brain damage.

Damage to the language (speech) area of the dominant cerebral hemisphere may be due to contusion or haemorrhage from a closed head injury, compression from a depressed fracture or direct trauma from a penetrating wound.

A severe closed head injury usually causes generalised effects with concussion and the associated shearing strains may damage the brain stem. On the other hand a penetrating wound causes direct focal damage, and although there is often some concussion as well, this may be minimal so that focal damage is occasionally sustained with no loss of awareness nor amnesia.

An example of this was a soldier who sustained a wound of the left Rolandic region in November 1944 causing transient motor aphasia, weakness of the right side of the face and numbness of the right arm; he remembered the wound and remained fully conscious. His legs were not affected and after being wounded he walked two miles to meet the stretcher-bearers. Bone fragments and damaged brain were removed at operation and he made a good recovery. Some years later he was killed in an accident and Fig. 10 showed the position of the brain wound.

If damage is confined to the speech area, dysphasia may be the only deficit; other focal signs may also occur in isolation or in combination, according to the site and extent of damage.

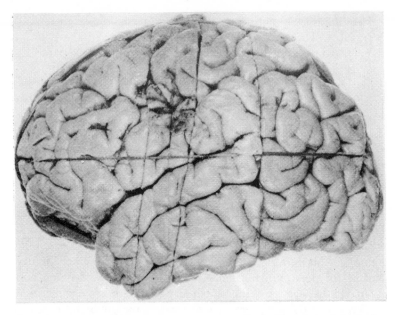

Fig. 10 Appearance of brain at postmortem. (From *Traumatic Aphasia*, by W. Ritchie Russell and M.L.E. Espir (1961). University Press, Oxford.)

Missile wounds may cause extensive damage, either due to indriven fragments of bone or haemorrhage. These may be fatal but, if not, the wound may be complicated by infection and abscess formation. Neurosurgical treatment is required to remove debris, pus, blood clots, bone fragments and the penetrating missile if accessible. *Posttraumatic epilepsy* is liable to develop in approximately 50% of such cases; this risk is very small in cases of closed head injury, especially when there is not a depressed fracture nor intracranial haematoma, and when the posttraumatic amnesia is relatively short (i.e. less than 24 hours).

Widespread brain damage usually causes prolonged coma. Eventual recovery of consciousness may then be accompanied by dementia sometimes with severe motor, sensory or visual deficits. Maximum recovery usually occurs during the first 1½–2 years after the injury, but disability—including dysphasia—is permanent in some cases. Speech therapy is indicated for dysphasia as soon as the patient can cooperate after the acute effects of the head injury, and should continue so long as progress is being made.

Intensive care units with specialised facilities for resuscitation have led to the survival of many young patients with severe head injuries. The extent of the brain damage and longterm prognosis is often difficult to determine initially, and occasionally intensive care leads to dramatic recoveries. Inevitably some tragic cases will remain severely disabled and require prolonged, possibly permanent, nursing or special social care.

Diffuse bilateral cerebral damage may cause dysarthria as part of a pseudobulbar palsy. In other cases dysarthria results from damage to the brain stem or cerebellum due to torsion with tearing of nerve fibres and haemorrhages.

Fractures of the base of the skull can cause tearing of the arachnoid mater, with leakage of cerebrospinal fluid (CSF) via the nose or ear (CSF rhinorrhoea and otorrhoea respectively). The tear can allow entry of pathogenic organisms with infection leading to meningitis and sometimes intracranial abscess formation. Fractures of the base of the skull may also cause damage to one or more of the cranial nerves. The filaments of the olfactory nerves traversing the cribriform plate in the anterior fossa of the skull may be torn and anosmia (loss of the sense of smell) is not an uncommon complication of severe head injuries, and sometimes occurs in this way even when there is no fracture. Occasionally the optic nerves or chiasm are damaged, and fractures of the petrous temporal bone are particularly liable to damage the acoustic or facial nerves, causing deafness or facial palsy (of LMN type) on the affected side. Damage to the vestibular mechanism, particularly the labyrinth, causes vertigo. During recovery this tends to be aggravated for some time by changes of posture, so-called *positional vertigo*. Although this usually subsides spontaneously, it is often troublesome for several months or more. This may be part of a *post-traumatic syndrome*, associated with impairment of speech, memory and other intellectual faculties, together with changes in personality, mood and behaviour such as disinhibition. These may persist after severe head injuries especially when there has been frontal and temporal lobe damage. Other cases develop a *traumatic neurosis* in which the predominant symptoms are persistent headache, depression, anxiety and irritability. These patients also complain of inability to concentrate, forgetfulness and lethargy, and they often fail to resume work, but there are usually no objective physical signs. This condition may be associated with organic deficits, but it is usually encountered in those who have sustained relatively trivial head injuries causing no, or only brief, concussion and particularly when litigation is pending.

Most of the severe closed head injuries in civilian personnel result from road traffic accidents, especially in motor cyclists and car drivers, whereas penetrating wounds are the result of military action.

In children brain damage may occur during birth, or later as the result of 'non-accidental injuries'—the so-called 'battered baby syndrome'.

Intracranial haemorrhage. Due to traumatic rupture of blood vessels, it constitutes one of the most serious and often fatal complications of a head injury. Single or multiple haemorrhages of varying sizes occur in the substance of the brain, forming an intracerebral or intracerebellar haematoma, or within part of the ventricular system (i.e. intraventricular haemorrhage).

Bleeding may also take place directly into the subarachnoid space (i.e. *traumatic subarachnoid haemorrhage*). The blood then becomes mixed with the CSF which will be revealed if lumbar puncture is done. The clinical signs of subarachnoid haemorrhage are due to irritation of the meninges by the extravasated blood, so that there is meningism consisting of headache, neck stiffness and photophobia. In mild cases the bleeding stops spontaneously, the blood in the CSF is absorbed and recovery ensues.

A head injury can also cause haemorrhage into the subdural space due to rupture of the veins draining into the venous sinuses and the resulting collection of blood becomes sealed off to form a *subdural haematoma*. In the acute stages this may be associated with severe cerebral damage and a high mortality rate. In some cases a subdural haematoma increases in size more slowly so that after a few weeks or months following the head injury there are signs of compression of the brain with raised intracranial pressure. The diagnosis is sometimes difficult, as the history of a preceding head injury is not always obtained, but prompt investigation and neurosurgical treatment usually results in recovery.

Head injuries, particularly with skull fracture, sometimes damage the meningeal vessels and cause bleeding into the extradural space. This *extradural haemorrhage* may be rapidly fatal, but the diagnosis should be suspected if the head injury is followed by deterioration in the level of consciousness and dilatation of one or both pupils. Occasionally this occurs after a period of recovery following the initial concussion so that there is a 'lucid interval' before coma again supervenes. An emergency operation to remove the extradural collection of blood and relieve the brain compression is then essential.

Further Reading

RUSSELL W.R. & ESPIR M.L.E. (1961) *Traumatic Aphasia*. University Press, Oxford.

CHAPTER 20
PARKINSON'S DISEASE

Parkinson's disease or *paralysis agitans* was described by Dr James Parkinson in 1817 when his monograph entitled *An Essay on the Shaking Palsy* was published. The shaking of the limbs had been noticed by Galen (200 AD), but it was Parkinson's classical description of the peculiar character of the tremor together with the other distinguishing features of the disease that established it as a clinical entity.

Parkinson's disease is due to an idiopathic degeneration of nerve cells in the basal ganglia and particularly the substantia nigra which produce the neurotransmitter dopamine. The normal balance between inhibitory dopamine and excitatory acetylcholine is disturbed by the deficiency of dopamine and results in the Parkinsonian syndrome or parkinsonism. In some cases this is symptomatic (i.e. attributable to drugs, infection or other diseases—see later) but in the majority, the cause of the degeneration is not known and it is this idiopathic disorder which is called *paralysis agitans* or Parkinson's disease. It usually begins after the age of 50, although occasionally earlier, with increasing incidence in later life. It is slightly more common in males than females and runs a progressive course but often quite slowly. As a rule it is not hereditary or familial. About 80 000–100 000 people have the disease in the UK and it is common in all parts of the world.

The main features of the disease are tremor, impairment of movements (hypokinesia), slowness of movements (bradykinesia) and rigidity, but their order of development is variable. Initially there may be slight loss of facial expression with lack of blinking and general slowness of movements and the tremor may begin insidiously in one hand. The tremor is a rhythmic to and fro movement, often of the thumb and fingers aptly described as 'pill-rolling'. It is variable and most noticeable when the arm is relaxed (e.g. in the sitting position or when walking) and is increased by stress, but reduced or abolished temporarily by holding it or gripping something and it does not occur during sleep. The tremor may spread to involve both arms and legs, although it is often more marked on one side and it may also affect the head, jaw, lips and tongue. Although the tremor is characteristic of the disease and may be very obvious and embarrassing, it does not occur in all cases, and the slowness of movement and rigidity with difficulty initiating action is frequently the most disabling. This causes difficulty in getting up from a chair and turning round, the facial expression becomes fixed and mask-like, and there is a lack of gesture and associated movements. Eye movements are usually unaffected apart from impairment of convergence. In some cases blinking is infrequent but can be induced in time with repetitive tapping on the glabella, and in a few cases there is spontaneous blepharospasm (i.e. involuntary tonic closure of the eyelids).

Loss of finely coordinated movements interferes with dexterity for occupational and daily living activities; shaving, eating and dressing become more difficult and writing decreases in legibility and size (micrographia). There is a disturbance of balance and gait, posture becomes rather stooped and the limbs slightly flexed, the legs tend to shuffle along so that walking appears hurried (festinant) with *marche à petit pas*. There is a tendency to freeze because of the difficulty in starting to walk, but the patient then takes small hurried steps with the body stooped trying to catch up with the centre of gravity, being unable to stop when pushed forwards (propulsion) or backwards (retropulsion), yet able to step carefully over obstacles or along railway sleepers, or even run. The stiffness of the muscles causes an uneven jerky resistance to passive movements, referred to as cogwheel rigidity, and this aggravates the slowness of movements. Although there may be considerable delay and difficulty in performing and coordinating movements, there is no actual loss of power, the tendon reflexes are usually unaffected unless reduced by the rigidity, and the plantar responses remain flexor.

Speech is affected in the majority of patients with Parkinson's disease, and this becomes more obvious as the tremor, hypokinesia and rigidity involve all aspects of the speech mechanism. Inflexion and rhythm are impaired and characteristically the voice becomes monotonous and reduced in volume. Rigidity of the respiratory muscles makes it impossible to raise the voice or shout and sentences tend to fade. Dysphonia is the result of impaired control of the laryngeal and respiratory muscles, articulation particularly of consonants becomes defective causing a slurring dysarthria or dys-

arthrophonia. Rigidity of the vocal cords can be seen on laryngoscopy and a low pitched and occasionally tremulous voice is associated with faulty abduction and adduction and tremor of the vocal
cords. Hypernasality of speech also occurs in some patients due to
rigidity of the palate and failure of closure of the nasopharynx. The
difficulty in initiating movements makes patients slower to
respond, but then there may be an acceleration of speech with com-
pulsive repetition, words being uttered faster and faster (palilalia),
becoming increasingly indistinct and trailing away inaudibly.
Excessive salivation and difficulty in swallowing lead to dribbling
and slobbering which may be aggravated by tremor of the tongue
and lips.

As dysarthria increases, so speech may become unintelligible.
Usually the voice becomes weak and monotonous first, followed
by dysarthria and hypernasality, and then variations in the rate of
speech. Speech therapy can help to strengthen phonation and
control the rate of speech, and delayed auditory feedback has
helped patients with the festinating type of speech difficulty.

Parkinson's disease per se does not cause dementia, although in
the advanced stages when speech and reactions are severely
impaired, it may be difficult to exclude this, and in some cases there
may be more widespread degenerative changes with cortical
atrophy (see Chapter 13).

Other known causes of the Parkinsonian syndrome include drugs
(e.g. reserpine, phenothiazines) and other toxic substances (e.g.
carbon monoxide and manganese) which diminish dopaminergic
activity. The infection, encephalitis lethargica, which was pan-
demic after the First World War was responsible for many cases
which were called postencephalitic Parkinsonism. Some other rare
conditions have to be distinguished from Parkinson's disease,
having similar extrapyramidal features usually with rigidity and
hypokinesia but little if any tremor, e.g. Wilson's disease (see
Table 7), the Steele–Richardson–Olszewski syndrome (progressive supranuclear palsy) and the Shy–Drager syndrome (a form of
Parkinsonism with postural hypotension).

Treatment of Parkinson's disease is possible with various anti-
cholinergic drugs of which benzhexol (Artane) is most often used
with benefit. Amantadine (Symmetrel) was originally produced as
an antiviral drug and this occasionally relieves Parkinsonism for a
short time, but the most dramatic advance came with the introduc-

tion of levodopa. Its beneficial action is due to its conversion to dopamine by an enzyme (dopadecarboxylase) in the brain. Adverse effects occur if the levodopa is converted to dopamine before it reaches the brain, and so levodopa is usually given now in tablets called Sinemet or Madopar where it is combined with a drug which prevents the extracerebral decarboxylation of levodopa which is then not converted to dopamine until it reaches the brain. This enhances its beneficial effects and it reduces the side effects. Another drug with effects similar to levodopa is bromocriptine (Parlodel). Levodopa and bromocriptine may improve the clarity and loudness of speech, although they do not do so invariably. Treatment may be most effective when first given, but benefit tends to wear off after a few months or years. There may then be rapidly alternating phases of improvement and deterioration, the so-called on–off effect, and involuntary movements usually of choreic type (see page 67) may develop. This can also distort speech producing oro-buccolingual dyskinesia which interferes with articulation. There is rolling and protrusion of the tongue with lip-smacking and chewing movements which usually lessen or stop if the dose of levodopa is reduced.

Surgical treatment with a stereotactic procedure is now less commonly performed as drug treatment is always tried first and operation would only be considered for those in whom drug treatment has failed and who remain seriously disabled by tremor or rigidity, particularly on one side. The aim is to make a surgical lesion in the globus pallidus or the ventro-lateral nucleus of the thalamus or their connections.

If a patient with Parkinson's disease has a stroke, the hemiplegia abolishes the tremor on the affected side, a fact recorded by James Parkinson in his monograph. Although the cause of Parkinson's disease remains a mystery, the advances in understanding of the biochemistry of the basal ganglia encourage hope that further research will lead to the discovery of even more effective treatment.

Further Reading

CRITCHLEY E.M.R. (1981) Speech disorders of Parkinsonism: a review. *J. Neurol. Neurosurg. Psychiat.* **44**, 751–8.
PARKINSON J. (1817) *An Essay on the Shaking Palsy.* Whittingham and Ronald, London.

PERRY A.R. & DAS P.K. (1981) In *Research Progress in Parkinson's Disease*, eds.
   F.C. Rose & R. Capildeo. Pitman Medical, Tunbridge Wells.
ROCHE PRODUCTS LTD (1970) *Parkinson's Disease and the Parkinsonian Syndrome.*
   Roche, London.

CHAPTER 21
MOTOR NEURONE DISEASE

Motor neurone disease (MND) is a progressive disease of both upper and lower motor neurones of unknown cause. Involvement of upper motor neurones (UMNs) results in degeneration of (a) the corticobulbar tracts causing pseudobulbar palsy, and (b) the corticospinal (pyramidal) tracts causing spastic paraparesis or tetraparesis. Involvement of lower motor neurones (LMNs) results in degeneration of (c) the motor nuclei of the cranial nerves in the brain stem causing bulbar palsy, and (d) the anterior horn cells in the spinal cord causing muscular atrophy (amyotrophy)—see Table 18.

Table 18   Motor neurone disease.

Part affected	Progressive clinical syndrome
1 UMNs	
(a) corticobulbar tracts	pseudobulbar palsy
(b) corticospinal (pyramidal) tracts	spastic paraparesis or tetraparesis (lateral sclerosis)
2 LMNs	
(c) motor nuclei of cranial nerves in brain stem	bulbar palsy
(d) anterior horn cells in spinal cord	spinal muscular atrophy (amyotrophy)

Each of these components may be involved separately or in combination, with one or other predominating. For example, patients may have either *progressive bulbar palsy* or *progressive spinal muscular atrophy*, or features of both. The clinical syndrome resulting from the combination of (b) and (d) is known as *amyotrophic lateral sclerosis* (ALS). These terms are sometimes used as the diagnosis, instead of motor neurone disease, ALS being favoured especially in the USA. Since these forms may be only part of the neurological picture, we prefer 'motor neurone disease' as the generic name.

The prevalence is about 5 per 100 000, the disease usually starting between the ages of 50 and 70 although it can occur at any age. Males are affected more than females in the proportion of 1.5–1 and in rare instances the condition may be familial. Although the cause is unknown, the pathological process appears to be that of degeneration of motor neurones and their fibre tracts.

The initial signs may be unilateral, but the condition is almost invariably progressive, becoming bilateral and more or less symmetrical. The onset is gradual and the clinical picture depends on which motor neurones are affected first, whether they are upper or lower motor neurones or both. Commonly, weakness and wasting start in the small muscles of one hand, then the other, gradually becoming worse and more extensive, due to increasing involvement of the LMNs. When the LMNs are degenerating, *fasciculation* may be seen in the muscles; this looks like twitching or flickering in the affected muscles and characteristically is seen in the tongue in cases of progressive bulbar palsy. When the UMNs forming the corticospinal tracts are involved, the tendon reflexes are increased and the plantar responses extensor. If there is coincidental involvement of the anterior horn cells (i.e. LMNs) the muscles waste and the reflexes become depressed or absent. Sensory loss does not occur, the intellect is not affected, and bladder and bowel control are retained.

Pseudobulbar palsy consists of dysarthria, dysphonia and dysphagia (difficulty in swallowing), with increased jaw, facial, palatal and pharyngeal reflexes. The tongue is spastic and moves slowly, and speech becomes slow and slurred. Not infrequently there is also emotional lability, and pathological laughing and crying may occur inappropriately without corresponding change in mood.

Patients with progressive bulbar palsy also have dysarthria, dysphonia and dysphagia, but with wasting and fasciculation of the tongue which appears wrinkled. Speech becomes increasingly slurred; the bilabial plosives—'p' and 'b' and the phonemes requiring lip rounding and spreading are affected due to weakness of the orbicularis oris muscle, and this also causes difficulty in whistling. The voice becomes weaker and monotonous due to laryngeal palsy. This dysphonia is aggravated by weakness of the respiratory musculature (i.e. the intercostal muscles and diaphragm) which also causes shortness of breath (dyspnoea). The soft palate may become immobile causing speech to have a nasal quality (hyperrhinolalia) due to nasal escape of air. Swallowing becomes increasingly difficult and is accompanied by reflux of fluids through the nose and drooling of saliva. Choking may also occur due to fluids or food going down the wrong way when swallowing. With weakness of the jaw muscles, biting and chewing become difficult and eventually the jaw droops.

The disease is usually fatal within 4 years of the onset, but when progressive bulbar and pseudobulbar palsy occur early, death may ensue within 2 years. Some cases of progressive spinal muscular atrophy, however, have survived for more than 10 years.

No specific treatment is available for the condition. With dysphagia, semi-solid foods like porridge and purees are usually easier to swallow than solids or liquids. Some patients are helped by cricopharyngeal myotomy, if lips and tongue movements are adequate to initiate swallowing.

The disturbance of speech may be an early sign of the disease. At first the voice tires easily and becomes rasping, later monotonous and nasal. Eventually the patient can make only inarticulate noises. Letter and word cards or a specially adapted electric typewriter may help, and a range of communication aids are now available for patients whose speech becomes severely affected. They should be supplied before speech becomes unintelligible. They may only be required for a short time until the terminal phase of the illness is reached, but they can reduce the terrible psychological burden that accompanies anarthria and allow at least some form of communication, especially as intellect is preserved to the end. A few exceptional patients have communicated by blinking in morse-code or by shining a light attached to their forehead on phrases on a screen.

Further Reading

CARROW E., RIVERA V., MAULDIN M. *et al* (1974) Deviant speech characteristics in motor neurone disease. *Arch. Otolaryngol.* **100**, 212–18.

PERRY A.R. (1982) *What can the Speech Therapist offer in Motor Neurone Disease?* In *Research Progress in Motor Neurone Disease*, ed. F.C. Rose. Pitman Medical, Tunbridge Wells.

PERRY A.R., GAWEL M. & ROSE F.C. (1981) Communication aids and patients with motor neurone disease. *Br. Med. J.* **282**, 1690–2.

ROSE F.C. (1977) *Motor Neurone Disease.* Pitman Medical, Tunbridge Wells.

CHAPTER 22
MULTIPLE SCLEROSIS

Multiple sclerosis (MS) is the commonest neurological disease affecting young adults in the UK. The prevalence varies in different parts of the world, being very low in the tropics and commoner in temperate climates with a tendency for clusters of cases to occur in certain areas. In England the prevalence is 50–80 per 100 000, rising to 127 per 100 000 in North-East Scotland and 300 per 100 000 in the Shetlands and Orkneys. Immigrants who have spent their childhood in countries with a low or high prevalence seem to carry their susceptibility from their country of origin. In spite of a great deal of research, the cause remains a mystery.

The axon (the central conducting part of the nerve fibre) is insulated by a surrounding sheath of myelin and the disease, MS, is characterised by patchy destruction of this sheath resulting in plaques of demyelination in the central nervous system (CNS). Initially there is an inflammatory or allergic reaction which subsides but damages the myelin leaving the axons intact. This process may recur in the same area and become more extensive or involve other parts of the CNS. Hardening of the plaques with time results in patches of sclerosis (scarring) and eventual degeneration of axons. Plaques may be scattered (disseminated) throughout the CNS, but they seem to have a predilection for certain parts (i.e. the optic nerves, cerebellum, brain stem and spinal cord). They may also occur in the cerebral hemispheres, not infrequently in the later stages of the disease, and particularly in the periventricular regions.

The disease usually starts in young adults between the ages of 20 and 40, but occasionally in the late teens and also in middle age. Females are affected more than males in the ratio of 3:2, and there seems to be a weak genetic influence, 5–6% of cases being familial. The genetic susceptibility to MS may be partly explained by a common but not exclusive association with certain HLA-linked genes. However, only a few of the close relatives carrying the same gene develop the disease, so that other genetic, environmental and immunological influences are considered likely to be important factors in the pathogenesis.

The mode of onset is variable and the course unpredictable. In some patients the initial symptoms reflect a single lesion and the diagnosis may be difficult; in others there is early evidence of two or more lesions, and special investigations may confirm the diagnosis. Typically the disease is characterised by relapses and remissions, but in about 20% of cases, particularly those starting after the age of 40, the disease is progressive. The first plaque may develop in an optic nerve (optic neuritis) causing pain and blurring or loss of vision in one eye. There is usually a spontaneous gradual recovery and remission may last for days, months, years or even indefinitely. A further episode (relapse) may occur at any time and involve another part of the nervous system (e.g. a plaque in the spinal cord causing weakness and sensory disturbance in one or both legs). Plaques occur either singly in various parts of the nervous system at different times, or in crops about the same time. Recovery from each relapse may take several weeks or months, but transient symptoms such as weakness, ataxia, paraesthesiae or blurring of vision may occur particularly in the early stages, and may be precipitated by stress, a hot bath, certain movements or exertion. Occasionally stereotyped repetitive paroxysmal disturbances including trigeminal neuralgia are troublesome. In some cases the course from the outset is relentlessly progressive, whereas in others deterioration follows later due to gradual extension and spread of the demyelinating process. In some cases fatigue is a prominent symptom. However, MS does not invariably result in severe disability; in a higher proportion than is generally realised —possibly 50% of cases—the course is relatively benign and the long-term prognosis is good in that there is little or no permanent restriction of employment or of other activities. In others after each successive relapse, there tends to be less recovery and thus more severe and persistent disability.

Plaques involving the cerebellum or its connections with the brain stem cause a variety of cerebellar signs which may include nystagmus, titubation (incoordinate movements of the head and neck) clumsiness of the hands with intention tremor and ataxia of gait. Speech becomes slurred, typically with a scanning or staccato type of dysarthria (see page 71). Manifestiations of the disease affecting other parts of the nervous system are frequently present at the same time or occur in subsequent relapses. These include visual and sensory symptoms, vertigo, loss of bladder control and upper motor neurone signs due to plaques in the spinal cord. Although plaques may also occur in the cerebral hemispheres, dysphasia is uncommon in MS.

The natural anxiety resulting from the unpredictable nature of the disease and uncertainty about the future, as well as any persistent disability, lead to depression which is the commonest affective disturbance in patients with MS. Nevertheless many patients remain outwardly cheerful and stoical, whereas pathological cheerfulness (euphoria), contrary to classical reports, is relatively rare. Euphoria, however, may accompany dementia, usually in the later stages when there is already severe physical disability. However, intellectual impairment is not a frequent problem and there should be increasing awareness of the large proportion of benign cases in which working capacity is not seriously affected.

The diagnosis of MS may be supported by finding abnormalities in the CSF, in particular a raised gammaglobulin level with a relative increase in the IgG fraction. Visual evoked responses may also help with the diagnosis, as abnormalities with a prolonged latency may indicate a subclinical attack of optic neuritis, and auditory evoked responses may show evidence of a brain stem lesion and so help to confirm the diagnosis in difficult cases.

There is as yet no specific cure for MS, but treatment of an acute episode with ACTH or steroids, starting as soon as possible following relapse, sometimes accelerates recovery. This treatment is usually continued for 1–4 weeks; more prolonged courses are not likely to help and are best avoided. Symptomatic measures to counteract depression, relieve spasticity and aid bladder control, as well as prompt treatment of any intercurrent infection are also very important. During periods of disability, physiotherapy is usually advocated and is often beneficial.

In view of evidence suggesting that a disorder of the body's immune reactions may contribute to the demyelinating process, various drugs and regimes which influence the immune mechanisms have been tried. These methods require complicated control, they are not free from risk and so far the results have been disappointing. It has also been found that the serum and brain levels of polyunsaturated fatty acids (PUFAs) are reduced in patients with MS, so that supplements of PUFAs, e.g. sunflower seed oil and 'Naudicelle' (a proprietary preparation containing a mixture of bio-oils including gamma-linolenic acid) have been recommended, together with various diets. There have been reports of slight reduction of relapse rates compared with controls but on the whole there has been little clear-cut or longterm benefit.

Further Reading

McAlpine D., Lumsden C.E. & Acheson E.D. (1972) *Multiple Sclerosis: a Reappraisal*, 2e. Churchill Livingstone, Edinburgh.

Matthews W.B. (1978) *Multiple Sclerosis—The Facts*. University Press, Oxford.

Millar J.H.D. (1971) *Multiple Sclerosis: A Disease Acquired in Childhood*. C.C. Thomas, Springfield, Illinois.

INDEX